MW01680379

Apollo's Creed

The story of our fight for time

A battle of love against cancer...

by Deb Estes

Cover Design
by Barbara Greene

A Books To Believe In Publication

Proudly Published in the USA by
Thornton Publishing, Inc
17011 Lincoln Ave. #408
Parker, CO 80134

Phone: (303)-794-8888
Fax: (720)-863-2013

www.BooksToBelieveIn.com/ApollosCreed.php

www.ProfitablePublishing.net
publisher@profitablepublishing.net

ISBN: 0-9779960-8-5

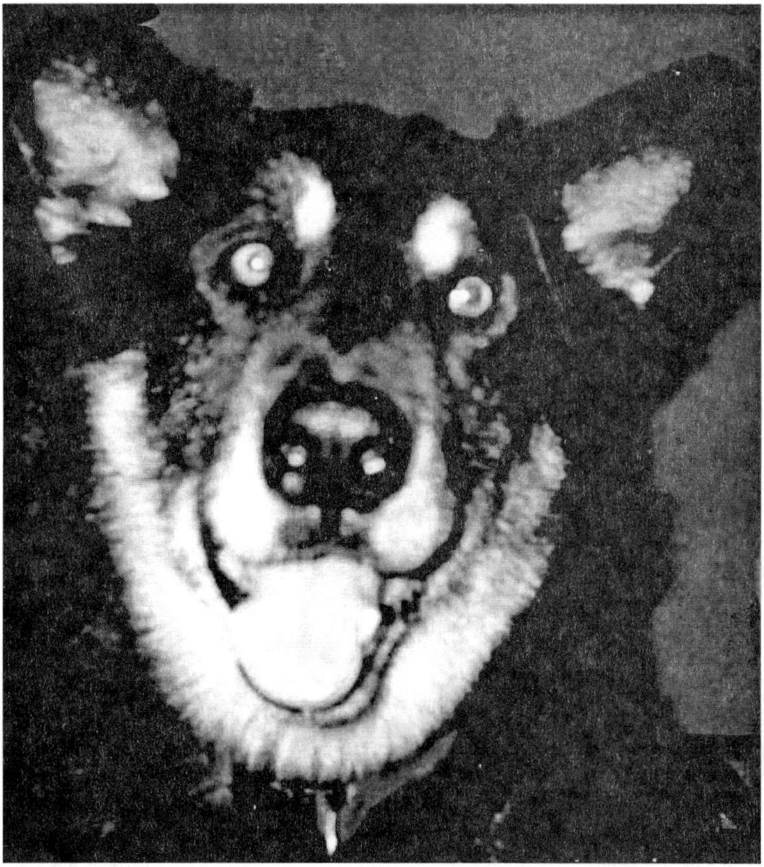

Contents

If You Can...

If you can start the day without caffeine,
If you can get going without pep pills,
If you can always be cheerful ignoring aches and pains,
If you can resist complaining and boring people with your troubles,
If you can eat the same food every day and be grateful for it,
If you can understand when your loved ones are too busy to give you any time,
If you can overlook it when those you love take it out on you when, through no fault of yours, something goes wrong.
If you can take criticism and blame without resentment,
If you can ignore a friend's limited education and never correct him,
If you can resist treating a rich friend better than a poor friend,
If you can face the world without lies and deceit,
If you can conquer tension without medical help,
If you can relax without liquor, if you can sleep without the aid of drugs,
If you can say honestly that deep in your heart you have no prejudice against creed, color, religion, or politics,

Then, my friend, you are almost as good as your dog.

~Author Unknown

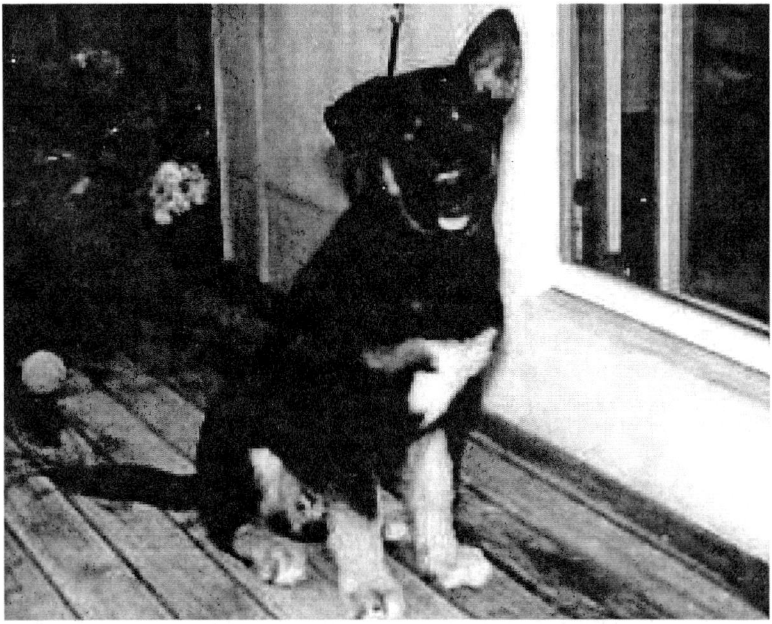

Foreword

Cancer happens.

Malignant cancers crash across all the lines of goodness, fairness, faith, love, 'quality of life' and ultimately life itself. Apollo's journey through malignant cancer, hand in paw, is the poignant story of a loving owner, dog and their battle to achieve quality of life for both of them. Apollo speaks through the eyes and emotions of his loving companion as she passionately describes her compelling drive and urgency to help them both, unconditionally. As it turns out, Apollo's creed of life becomes focused upon both his and her "quality of life."

With unspoken determination 'he' becomes the teacher "teaching" that cancer is not about dying but learning to live the best life possible. Apollo "teaches" that the "will to live" is a powerful force.

At the same time the dynamics of bonding and spiritual attachment become powerfully defined. The patient and the caretakers work feverishly to gain an understanding of the mechanisms of disease and the properties of healing: mentally and physically. Loud and clear, from compassionate touches to the pursuit of learning, the patient and his devoted owner experience a deepening and ever widening bond of love and compassion.

~H.C. (Doc) Gurney, D.V.M.

Apollo's Creed

Introduction

Some people believe angels have wings. This is a true story about an angel with four legs and a fur coat. It is a story about the lessons in life I learned from my best friend, my constant companion, my dog Apollo—lessons learned about life, love, spirit, compassion, courage, hope, determination, persistence, laughter, loyalty, happiness and being a better person. This is also about allowing the most important chapter in my life to close with peace, love, acceptance, and without regret.

I am not an accomplished author, nor an experienced writer; I am simply a dog owner who shared life with a best friend, my dog Apollo, for ten and a half years.

My four-legged friend and I were inseparable. Every time we moved into a new neighborhood we were immediately known, and commonly referred to, as "the girl with the big dog."

Apollo accompanied me to the grocery store, dry cleaners, bank, on wintertime sales calls, and the annual Christmas tree shopping expedition. Apollo and I visited every park in south metro Denver and shared pleasure trips across Colorado from Durango to Aspen. Apollo wasn't *just a dog*, he was my best friend, and in many senses we grew up together.

I am writing this book to share our story with other pet owners. I hope that this book will provide some advice, strength, comfort and support to pet owners who find themselves faced, as I was, with the imminent loss of their best friend.

I hope to help pet owners handle the care of their best friends in both life and death. Our story will provide some resources, treatment options and finally, some ways to say goodbye.

When we experience such a strong bond with our pet, they are not merely a pet, but rather a family member, and to say the loss of our beloved friend is difficult is an understatement. Psychologists have found when we have a strong bond with pets that are

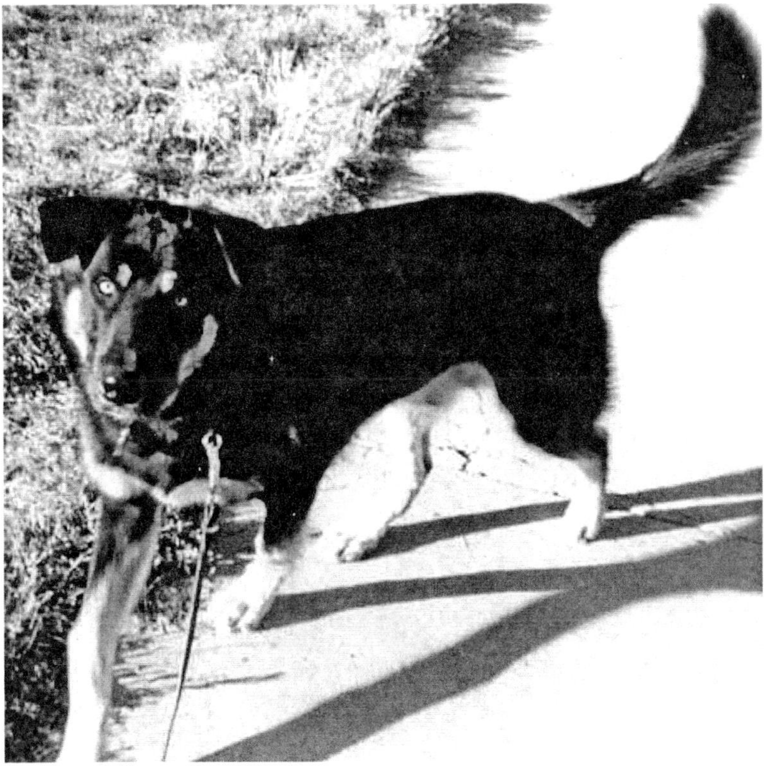

family members, their death results in the same feelings of grief and emotions associated with a close human's death. I believe that in some cases the grief may be felt to an even greater extent, perhaps because some people do not understand how much friendship we share with a close pet, leaving us very much alone in the grieving process.

The vast amount of emptiness left by Apollo's death will never be filled. By telling Apollo's and my story, I hope pet owners will realize that they are not alone in the feelings they have for their companion. I will provide some empowerment, encouragement and resources in dealing with a pet's illnesses and coping with an eventual and overwhelming loss.

It is only with the love and support of family and close friends, and knowing that without a doubt I did absolutely everything humanly possible to take care of Apollo, especially in his last challenging year of life, that I find comfort.

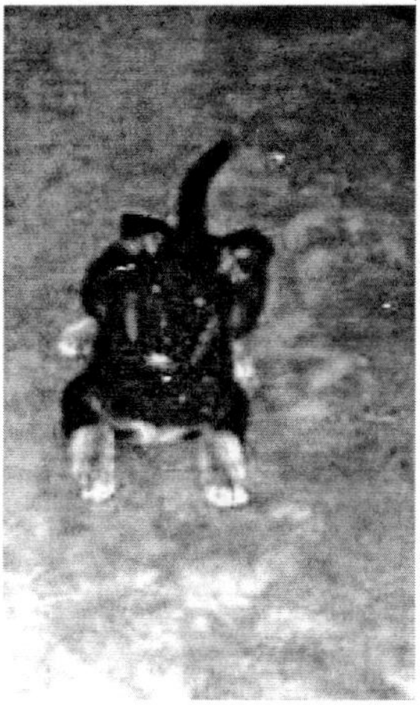

Chapter 1

A Happy Dog, A Routine Walk, Our Life Would Never Be the Same

It was Friday, December 13th a night I will never be able to forget. Around 9:30 that evening my husband, Joe asked me if I was ready to take Apollo for his nightly walk.

Just two evenings before, Joe, Apollo and I had gone out and chosen our Christmas tree. This was the annual Christmas tree shopping trip for Apollo; Apollo and I shopped for the "perfect" tree together for nine years.

Joe and I had just finished stringing the lights on the tree we had brought home a couple of nights earlier. I thought I would do a little more decorating, so Joe and Apollo went for a walk without me that night.

I added a few ornaments to our Christmas tree, cleaned up the mess we had left from the lights and decided to call it a night. After all we had the rest of the weekend to finish our Christmas decorating.

I went to fetch Apollo's dog bowl and filled it with his ice cubes and treats, walked upstairs and placed it on the floor at the foot of the bed. This was our usual bedtime routine, but this would turn out to be an unusual night.

I heard the front door open a little later, and knew Apollo would be bounding upstairs looking for his bedtime snack any minute. Apollo ran to the kitchen first looking for me and his treats. I could hear him scurrying about on the hardwood floors downstairs. When he didn't find what he was looking for downstairs, he knew he would find his treats upstairs in his usual place.

He was scurrying across the hardwood floors and as he rounded the corner to race up the stairs what I heard next I will NEVER be able to forget.

I heard Apollo's paws hit the carpet on the way up the stairs followed by an excruciating yelp and then a dull thud. I was out of bed and downstairs in a less than a second. There at the bottom of the stairs in a heap, lay a whining Apollo. As tears began rolling down my cheeks, I asked Joe what happened. He said that the moment Apollo's back legs hit the carpet on the stairs Apollo's right back leg snapped and broke. Joe told me he actually heard Apollo's bone snap.

Joe had advanced first aid training and had been on the ski patrol for years. As a result, he had seen many broken bones. But I couldn't believe it. I kept asking "Are you sure? Are you sure? How is that possible? How could have Apollo possibly broken his leg so easily?" But after checking Apollo, I was sure Joe was right.

Joe and I sat on the floor next to Apollo just stunned! Neither one of us wanted Apollo to move;

nor did we want to move. It was almost 11:00 p.m. and after about 20 minutes I got up off the floor and went to phone our veterinarian. The office answering service picked up and provided the regular office hours and said that in case of an emergency after hours go to an emergency veterinary clinic. Joe asked me if I wanted to take Apollo to an emergency veterinary clinic, but after thinking about it for a few minutes I had to say, "No." I just didn't know that I felt comfortable taking Apollo to a clinic he had never been to before, and to get treated by a stranger.

Apollo was a big dog. Ironically one time his veterinarian and I actually discussed how bad it would be if he did ever break a bone. She had told me that just due to his size it would be a horrible situation.

When I asked Joe what he thought an emergency clinic would do he said he felt that they might just give Apollo some pain killers and keep him until the morning when we could take him to his regular veterinarian, or he said, they might just want to put him down depending on the severity of the break.

By this time, it was almost midnight and Apollo had stopped whining and was starting to fall asleep. I decided that since Apollo was going to sleep and he probably wouldn't be getting up attempting to walk, he would be better off being comfortable and seeing his regular veterinarian in the morning. I knew that I would be able to reach his veterinarian's office by 7:30 or 8:00 a.m. Saturday which meant only seven and a half hours away from being in familiar hands.

I didn't want Apollo to be alone through the night, so Joe and I grabbed some blankets and some pillows; I slept on the floor with Apollo just to make sure he was okay. I refused to leave Apollo alone because I was afraid he would wake up during the middle of the night and try to come upstairs for his bowl of treats and only make his broken leg worse.

I was not about to let Apollo down, so while Joe stayed with him I brought down the bowl of treats and ice cubes that Apollo had expected every night for the last nine years. I had given Apollo three aspirin just in case he was in pain. I wouldn't have chosen to wait until morning, but once he had the aspirin, Apollo didn't seem to be in any pain.

I elevated his broken leg on several pillows so that it was level with his body, put a pillow on the floor for myself, threw several blankets over both of us, snuggled up to Apollo and scratched his chest. Before long Apollo was sound asleep and seemed to be resting comfortably. I lay absolutely still listening to each tick of the clock, hoping and praying that morning would come soon.

At 7:30 Saturday morning, I quietly got up, trying hard not to disturb Apollo and got to the phone. I called our veterinarian's office and left a message that Apollo had broken his leg and we wanted to get him in as soon as possible. Unfortunately, when I got up to make the phone call, Apollo also tried to get up, yelped and then limped over to me on three legs. All I could do was hug him and promise him that we were going to fix everything very soon. Within a few minutes I received a call back from our veterinarian's office telling us to bring Apollo right in.

Joe thought about how we were going to get Apollo transported to the veterinarian's office. He said that we needed to immobilize Apollo and keep him off his broken leg. He asked one of our neighbors if we could borrow their Jeep and went to another neighbor and asked if he could come over and help us lift Apollo into the Jeep. We gently placed Apollo on an ironing board and used wide elastic belts to wrap him to the board to keep him from moving.

This was difficult because poor Apollo didn't understand what was happening and he kept trying to get up. We were trying to do the best thing for Apollo. I was relieved that Joe and I hadn't tried to lift and carry him out the night before without any help; it might have only made the break worse.

I rode in the back of the Jeep with Apollo on the drive to his veterinarian assuring him that he would be okay. It was the longest 15 minute drive of my entire life. I told my doggie as I petted him that I would take good care of him. He knew and trusted exactly that; after all he had been my very special dog since the day we first met. I would do what was best for my best pal.

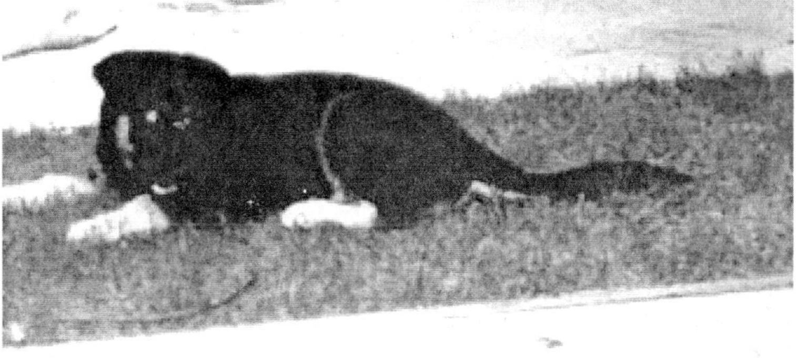

Chapter 2

From the Beginning This Was A Very Special Puppy Dog

As I look back to the beginning when Apollo came into my life and I distinctly remember I thought about getting a dog. For the very first time since my college days I wasn't working more than one job and I didn't have family living anywhere nearby. I had friends who had dogs and I found myself "dog sitting" often and enjoying the "job" very much. A very good friend of mine had a German Shepherd expecting a litter of puppies in July of that year.

I had grown up with German Shepherds, so I knew they made great pets. I also really liked Newfoundland and St. Bernards, but I was living in a townhouse and didn't have much of a yard for such a large breed of dog. So, I thought I would probably wait for one of the shepherd pups. I really just wanted a dog to love and spoil, and always have around.

Another one of my friends heard I was thinking about a puppy and she had a friend who had a litter of German Shepherd/Alaskan Malamute puppies ready for new homes. I set out to just look and to see some puppies similar to what I would be looking for a few months down the road.

This litter of puppies was a cute little bunch and the owner had both the mother and the father. The father was a large, beautiful, almost solid black German Shepherd named Rex. The mother was a huge stunning Alaskan Malamute named Ginger. She was sweet, and very beautiful. The puppies were delightful and a playful mix. I had not even considered getting a puppy that day but I should have known better.

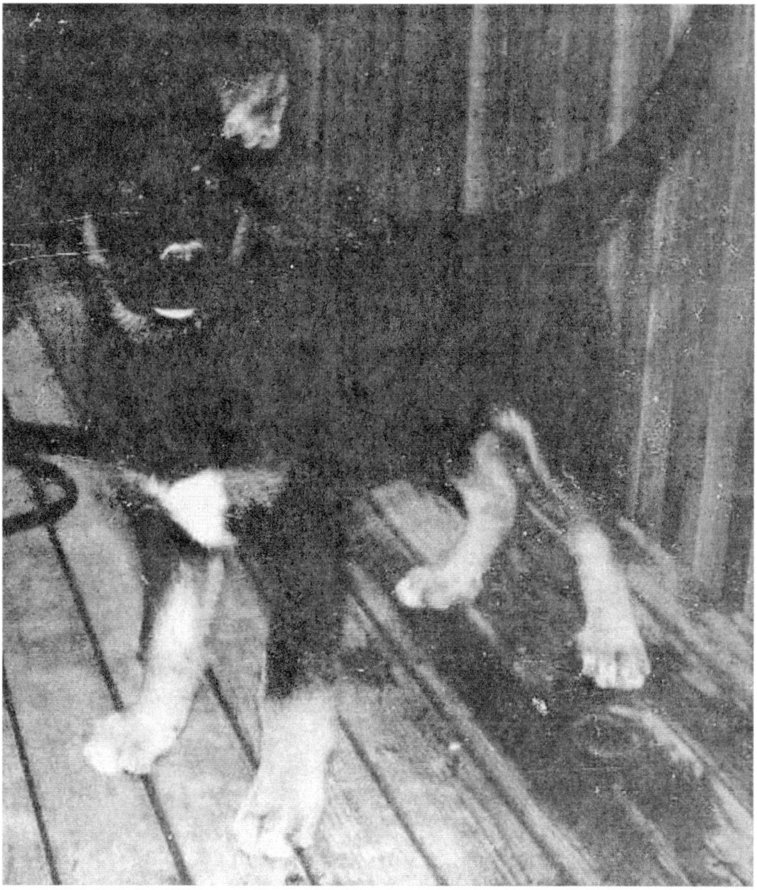

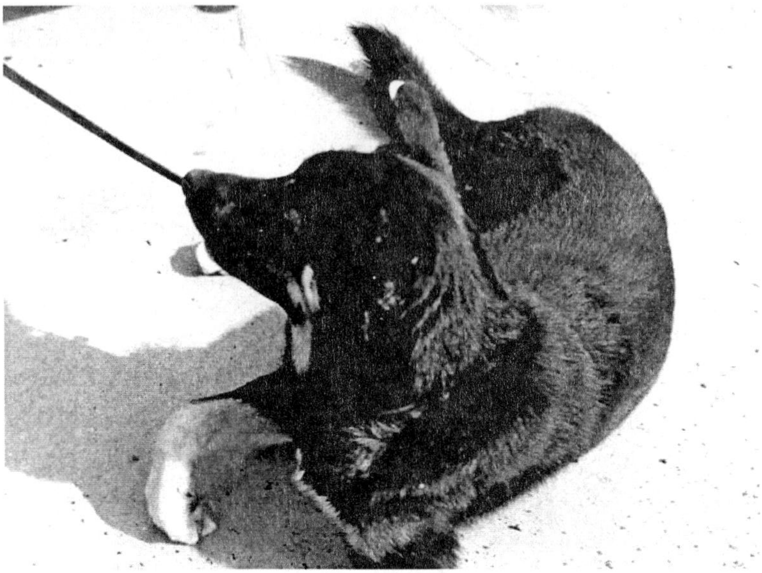

The shyest puppy of the litter caught my eye. While all of the other puppies jumped around and yapped for attention this puppy, even though he was the largest of the litter, went hiding behind the owner's couch apparently wanting to be an observer, rather than a player. He immediately grabbed my attention. He was the puppy who got my attention. He had the BIGGEST paws, definitely the largest puppy of them all, and he had big blond eyebrows that moved up and down with the movement of his eyes; he was the puppy I just had to have at that very minute, this puppy had won my heart.

I paid $50.00 for my mixed breed mutt who would later prove to be not only priceless but also irreplaceable.

I went home with my new puppy, totally unprepared. I had to stop at the grocery store on my way home to at least purchase some dog food so that I had something to feed him that night.

Within hours of bringing my puppy home, I named him "Apollo," after Apollo Creed, from the movie "Rocky." I thought it was the perfect name for this puppy. He had these HUGE paws and he seemed to be "jabbing" whenever he sat up. He was big, muscular and was almost all black except for the blond eyebrows and a white triangle on his chest. I knew that I had found the perfect puppy…my puppy! Apollo was the perfect name for him; later in his life he would prove he was indeed a true fighter.

The following morning I called my friend to let her know what I had done and let her know that I wouldn't be getting one of her German Shepherd pups. She advised me on what premium dog food I should purchase for the puppy and she explained kennel-training to house break Apollo. I was working a full-time job, and still paying off college loans, so like many young working adults I didn't have much extra money. I decided that a big box would serve as Apollo's kennel.

I was determined Apollo was going to be well trained and very obedient; no sleeping on the bed, no eating table scraps and I was going to be the master. Little did I know he would become the master, teaching me lessons about life no human ever could.

He was always a very good dog. He was well-mannered, had a mild temperament, great personality and was VERY strong willed, which probably helped him through his last and only health challenges.

Apollo and I set off on our first shopping expedition for all of the puppy items he absolutely needed. The first thing I heard when I carried Apollo (since I didn't even have a leash or collar yet) into the pet shop was, "that's going to be a BIG dog!" The owner of the pet shop just happened to have three German Shepherds and she said none of them ever had paws that big when they were puppies. I knew I had always wanted a big dog so I was happy to hear that. I wanted a dog to spoil and take care of so Apollo left the pet shop with toys, food, dog treats, and of course, a leash and collar.

That night, I put Apollo in his kennel (the big box) and he whined, cried and knocked it over. I smoothed out his blankets in the box, picked him up and gently put him back in his makeshift kennel with a wind-up alarm clock (I heard this was supposed to

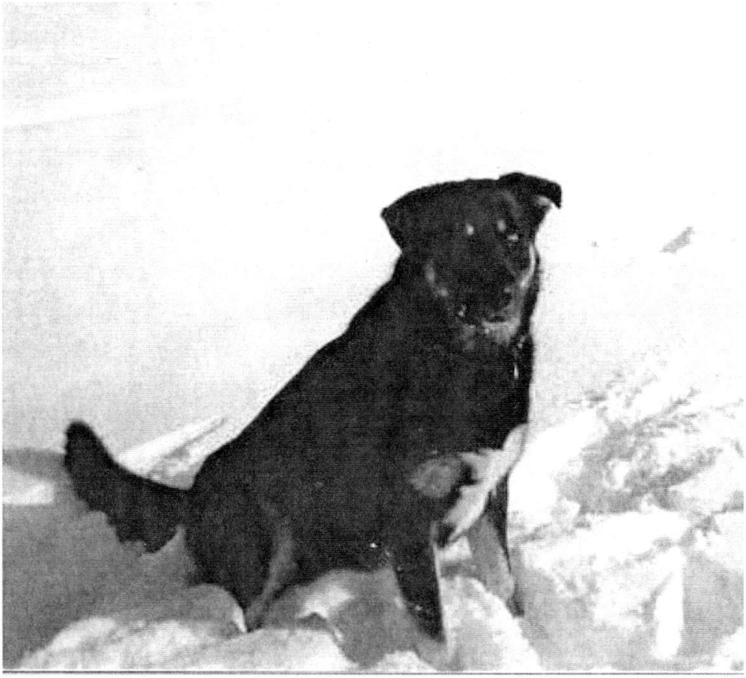

help him sleep). Apollo continued to cry and knocked over his sleeping quarters several more times. I was shocked that he could possibly keep knocking over this big box; he was definitely much stronger than I realized. He was nine weeks old and 19 pounds.

I had to wake up at 5:30 each morning, and I really needed to get some sleep so I began sleeping on the floor next to Apollo and his kennel, petting him constantly. As long as I kept petting him he slept quietly but if I stopped petting him, he immediately began to whine.

It was easy understand why, after a few nights of this routine, I decided to forget the make-shift kennel and take Apollo upstairs with me to sleep on the bed each night. It was then that Apollo and I began the tradition of taking a big bowl of ice cubes and dog treats upstairs each night at bedtime. After a while, it almost became a game for Apollo. He would sit patiently and watch me fix a bowl of ice cubes and treats, and when I said "bedtime," he would race upstairs and sit at the foot of the bed wagging his tail and then devour his treats. This became a nightly ritual we continued for the ten and a half years I had my puppy dog.

Although I had vowed Apollo would only have dog food and other acceptable dog treats, he was once again going to change my plan.

My parents and youngest brother had come to Denver to visit. One of my Dads' favorite appetizers was cold-boiled shrimp. My youngest brother, who was on his way to college had acquired a taste for cold beer. Between the two, Apollo never had to choose what he really wanted to eat...he had cold boiled shrimp, ice cold beer and grilled meat. He loved it all; so much for the strict canine diet.

Apollo was a happy dog and after all I said I wanted to have a dog to spoil. I figured some extra treats now and then wouldn't hurt him, so I enjoyed occasionally taking Apollo to a drive through burger place, where I would order him a cheeseburger, fries and a large cup of water. He even learned to drink from the to-go cup!

Apollo always sat in the front seat with me, with one front paw on my shoulder, his tail wagging enthusiastically, eager to smell the treats. When we were handed the food, I always heard, "That's a huge dog." When I told them "this food is for Apollo," he would often get a few extra fries from the window attendant.

When Apollo was five months old he weighed in at 50 pounds, and it wasn't puppy fat. He had a huge chest and a very large bone structure.

My good friend told me that I should probably start obedience training right away because Apollo was getting to be so big and she wanted to make sure I would have good control of him. So, we began our first obedience classes at Rocky Mountain Schutzand.

Most of the dogs there were German Shepherds, Dobermans or Rotweillers. Apollo was the only mixed-breed puppy, and he was definitely the largest in his age group. Apollo was extremely smart and learned very fast; when he wanted to. In addition to being physically strong, one of the instructors told me that Apollo was the most strong-willed dog he had ever worked with, and he had trained many, many dogs in obedience and protection for the Sheridan Colorado Police Department.

Part of Apollo's strong will was probably due to the fact that I wanted him to be a companion pet; not a show dog in obedience or protection. So, even though Apollo understood how to heel perfectly, when I took him on walks I didn't care if he wanted to investigate a fire hydrant or anything else that caught his attention.

I bought a 25 foot retractable leash so he could have a little freedom and yet I could still make sure he would not run out into the street.

I also learned at his training that he didn't like to be taken away from me to be worked or trained by any of the instructors.

Once, when one of the instructors tried to get Apollo to go with him, Apollo sat stubbornly looking first at me and then at the instructor as if to say "make me." The instructor tried to yank Apollo up from a sitting position. That was when I decided maybe we should try a different obedience school.

Our next obedience school went well but they rewarded good behavior and learning with treats. Apollo was rapidly approaching seven months and 70 to 75 pounds. The only real thing he hadn't mastered was walking off-leash, and I really wanted him to be able to go on a walk without one. I only weighed 105 pounds, so with Apollo still growing and gaining over ten pounds a month, it became evident that training with treats might not be our best option. I set out to find yet another style of obedience class.

The last and final obedience class focused on a lot of eye contact with dogs. Rewarding Apollo was accomplished with a lot of praise, love and attention. Ignoring Apollo was the way to show him that he was misbehaving. We almost passed this class, except for the walking without a leash, so it was a good thing someone invented a retractable leash. I also noticed that if I did ignore Apollo he immediately changed whatever he was doing in order to get my love and attention again. He was really very easy to train at this point. I think he must have been tired of "schools."

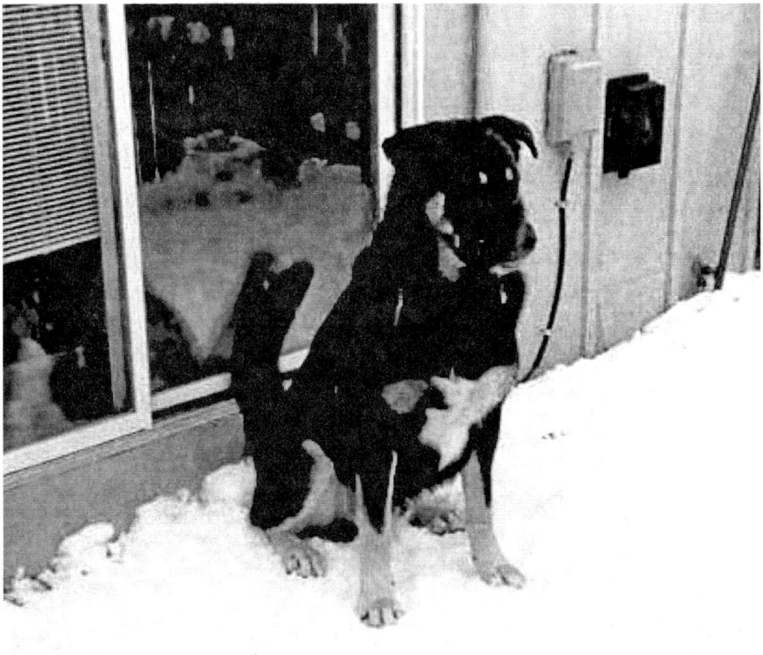

Chapter 3

My love, My Constant Companion & Protector

During Apollo's life, I worked in outside medical sales and had a remote office at home. If I wasn't on a sales call, I was in my office working on the phone and/or on the computer. Our routine was to go for a nice walk to the park in the mornings before I went into the office or left on sales calls. If I had an early flight to catch I always took Apollo for his morning

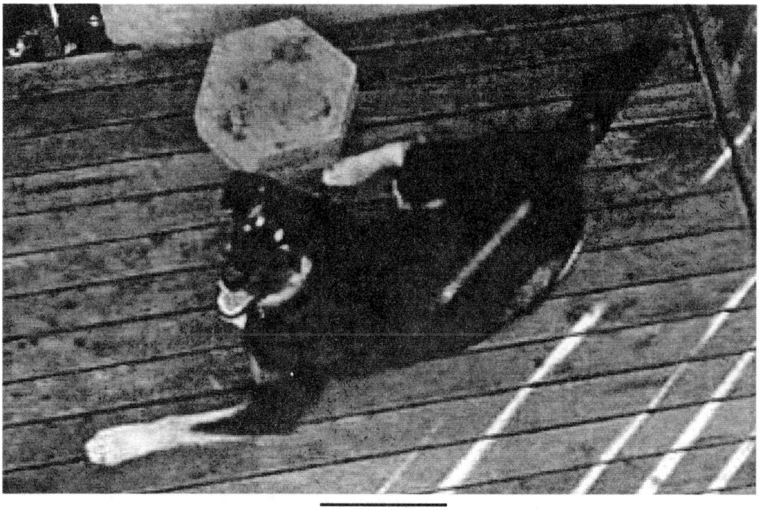

walks sometimes as early as 5:30. Once Apollo had his morning walk he was content to have a few dog treats and a rawhide chew and lay at my feet. He was a great office companion because he only barked when someone rang the doorbell and when he wanted to come inside.

Every night, I took Apollo for another nice long walk. He acted as if he knew what time it was and every night about 8:00 he would "talk" and hang out at the front door. This was different than if he just needed to go out or wanted to lay on the deck in the summertime, then he would sit at the back sliding glass door and paw the door to let me know he wanted to go outside. He never really asked for much, yet he gave me so much.

Once, when I had to drive to the western slope, I took Apollo with me. We stayed in Glenwood Springs, Colorado. I requested a room at the hotel with an outside entrance. No one even knew Apollo was there, and it was better than being alone because I had my best friend with me.

No matter where I went, as long as it wasn't too hot outside, Apollo went with me; he would rather have been waiting in the car than waiting home alone.

I drove a Saturn coupe with a sunroof and Apollo would sit in the front passenger seat with one paw on my shoulder and his head sticking out the sunroof...he definitely made some heads turn! During the hot summer months when I took Apollo with me, I locked one set of keys in the car with the air conditioner on and I took the other key with me to run into the dry cleaners or bank. One time, my neighbor walked by as I was getting back into my car with some doggie ice cream for Apollo. He remarked, "All Apollo needs now is a pair of sun glasses."

When Apollo was eight months old, I bought a German Shepherd puppy for my parents, but as it turned out, it wasn't quite the dog they were looking for. Because I was living in a rented townhouse I really didn't have enough space for two dogs so I called the Denver K-9 unit and offered to give them a dog. They sent the officer responsible for the K-9 unit to my house to take a look at the "volunteered" dog.

After the officer had been there observing the dogs for a little while he told me he definitely couldn't take my dog. At that point I hadn't told him which dog was really "my" dog. I asked why and he said of Apollo, "Because you and your dog have such a strong bond, he is great protection for you. If your dog heard fear or terror in your voice he would literally kill for you." I found that hard to believe because Apollo was so friendly with everyone we met and he had never displayed any sign of being the least bit aggressive. The officer told me that while observing us, Apollo never lost sight of me, and that as long as I was okay with people and what was going on around us, Apollo would be fine. However, if I were ever in danger, Apollo would be the best protection I could have. I think that was the first time I ever thought about Apollo being my protector.

I was more than relieved that the officer didn't choose to take Apollo, because I never wanted to give Apollo up. My thought had been that the K-9 unit would want the purebred German Shepherd. As it turned out, the K-9 unit couldn't take the German Shepherd either, because she had pancreatitis. I did a lot of searching and found her a wonderful home with lots of space to run so Apollo and I both took her to her new home.

After sharing his home for with another dog, Apollo once again had all the love and attention to himself. He had been patient, yet obviously spoiled as an only dog.

Apollo proved to be a great protector on one of our trips back from visiting my family in Durango, Colorado. We were driving through a small town hosting a big motorcycle rally complete with a large burley motorcycle group. I felt rather intimidated as

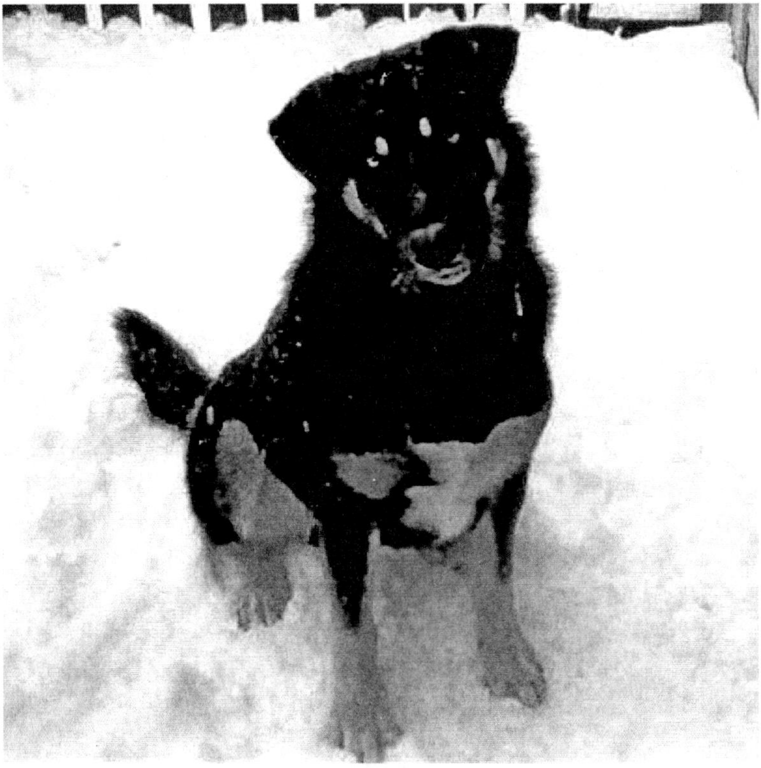

I was driving through the hundreds of cyclists lining the street. I called for Apollo. He had been lying down asleep in the back seat, and I said, "Come and jump up with me." He woke up, jumped to the front passenger seat, put one paw on my shoulder and put his head out the sunroof and I felt safe. Once we hit the interstate I stopped at the first place I found and bought Apollo a hamburger. He deserved it. Then I truly believed he was my protector.

During our years together I went back to college to earn my graduate degree. I felt terrible because I was in class two nights a week from six to ten, and I worked all day. Rather than leave Apollo at home alone during the winter I would take him with me. He waited contently, sleeping in the car with a bowl of ice cubes and dog treats and usually a nice big rawhide chew. I had three breaks each evening so I would let Apollo out of the car and take him for walks around the campus. I told Apollo he was probably the only dog who ever went to graduate school and didn't even have to pay tuition.

When I completed my graduate degree, six of my classmates and I had a celebration party at my house, with lots of barbecue and fixings, cold beer and champagne. Apollo was there and I made sure he had his share of all of the food. I considered Apollo a graduate too; he had been there with me all along the way! Apollo was my hero and he deserved the accolades and celebration too.

Chapter 4

We Became a Family Always Including Apollo

I met my husband to be in February. Our first few dates were tennis dates during that summer and we met at various tennis courts. Our first dinner date was in September and Joe picked me up at my home. Joe was a little surprised at exactly how big Apollo was, of course he had heard so much about Apollo,

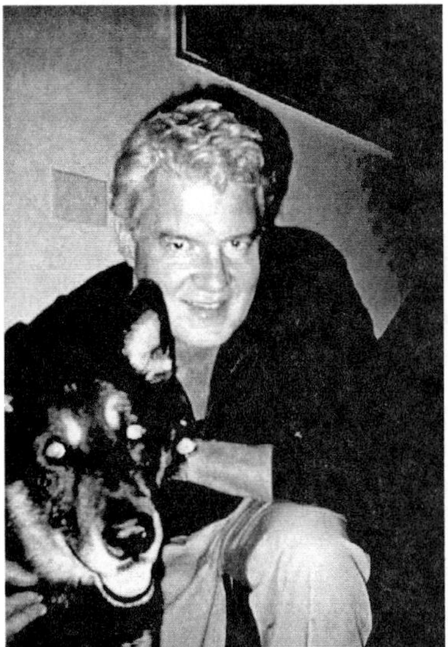

but until he actually saw him in person it was hard to imagine his size. Thankfully, he liked big dogs. Soon Joe and me, as well as Apollo, became inseparable.

After watching Monday night football and sharing pizza, Joe and I would take Apollo for his evening walk. Joe and Apollo became good friends and often before Joe and I would go out for an evening date we would take Apollo for a short walk before we left and again once we got back. During the snowy cold winter evenings, I became spoiled. If it was really cold outside Joe would take Apollo out for his walk and I would stay inside cozy and warm. When I would go over to Joe's house for dinner we would build a huge roaring fire in the fireplace and leave the door to his courtyard open so that Apollo

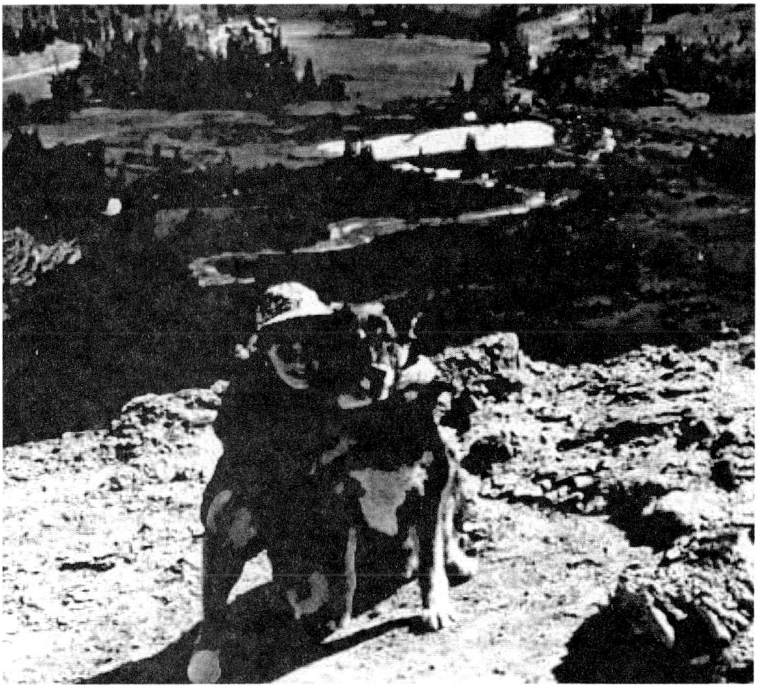

could enjoy the cool air and yet come in and be with us whenever he wanted. Joe also quickly realized when he had me over for dinner he was really cooking for three.

We drove to Durango for Christmas that year and of course took Apollo with us. Joe was very impressed at how easily Apollo traveled for the seven hour drive. I shared some of the memories I had taking Apollo with me to visit my family.

There was one Christmas when there was so much snow that I didn't want to drive to Durango, so I purchased an airline ticket and a large kennel for Apollo. The kennel was so big I had to take it apart to get it in my car. We drove up to the baggage drop off, I got out of the car, and had to put the kennel together before I could put Apollo in it and take him into the airport. When we returned, I ran to the parking lot, retrieved my car, went to pick Apollo up and did the same thing, only in reverse. I never once left Apollo behind when I went to visit my family.

There was only one time I had a problem with Apollo in Durango. I had let him off his leash on one of our walks. We were on a ranch, nowhere near a busy street, when, without warning, Apollo bolted. He ran right under a fenced coral with three horses inside! While Apollo seemed to be having the time of his life running around and up to the horses, I was in a panic. No matter how many times I called Apollo to come back, even when I was trying to show him I had really good treats for him, he was having too much fun with the horses to come back to me. After what seemed like an eternity, the owner of the horses spotted us and came to the rescue, rounding up the horses and leading them back to his barn. I was so relieved that Apollo hadn't been kicked, that all I could do was thank the kind gentleman and hug Apollo, even though I was furious with him. That was the last time I let Apollo off his leash until he was ten years old.

During the summer months when it became unbearably hot in Denver, Joe and I would leave on Sunday mornings for Vail, Colorado. It was only an hour and fifteen minutes from our doorstep to a beautiful location and at least 20 degrees cooler. Apollo loved walking along Gore Creek, and inevitably walking IN Gore Creek, enjoying the

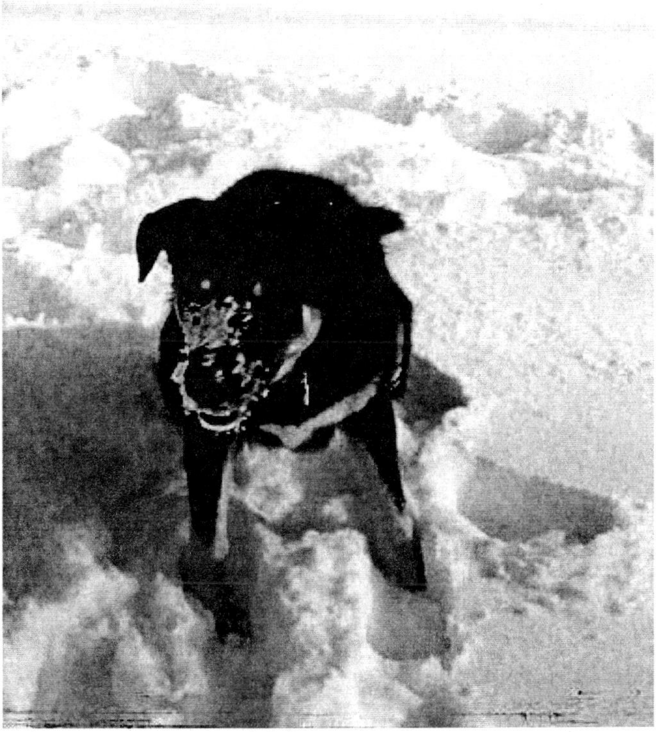

mountain, village and all of the attention he received. Almost everyone in Vail Village who saw us walking would come up to ask what kind of dog he was, could they pet him, what was his name and, of course, how much does he weigh? People were drawn to Apollo; he was like a giant teddy bear. Apollo loved the people and attention as much as they loved him. It usually took at least two and a half hours to walk from one end of Vail Village to Lionshead, at the other end of town. Without Apollo it would have taken about 20 minutes; apparently Apollo was not in any great hurry.

We usually ended our Sundays in Vail at Haagen Dazs ordering three ice cream cones; one plain vanilla for Apollo of course. All Apollo ever received

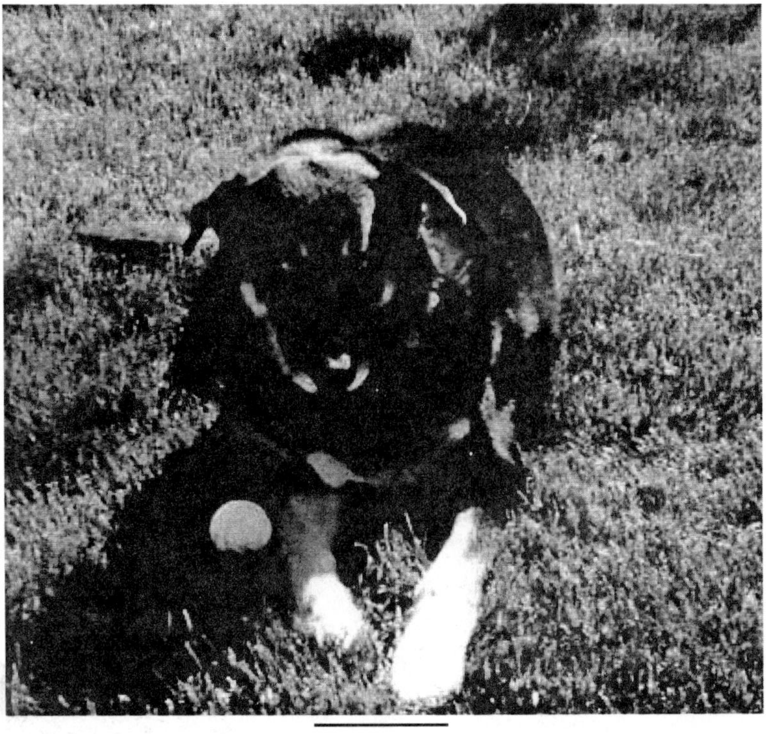

in his entire lifetime was kindness and compassion, and he only responded to people he met with gentleness and love. In all the years I had Apollo, he never once growled at another person. He treated everyone as if they were his friends, as long as it seemed okay with me.

In December of that year, Joe and I thought it'd be nice to spend our New Year's in Estes Park, Colorado. It was close to Denver, right on the edge of Rocky Mountain National Park. We thought it would be fun to take Apollo and go snowshoeing. We found a wonderful little rustic cabin, with a wood-burning fireplace, barbecue grill and a spectacular view. We spent one evening walking around Estes Park admiring the town's Christmas decorations, Apollo walking with us. Again, everyone who ran into us asked about Apollo and as usual he loved the attention.

The next evening we built a huge fire in the fireplace and opened the door so Apollo could go out on the deck and be cool and comfortable. After dinner we took another walk through a nearby mountain trail that Apollo loved as much as we did. Apollo really enjoyed being in the mountains.

During the fall, Apollo and I surprised Joe with a trip to Aspen for Joe's birthday. We had reservations at the well-known Little Nell Hotel. Dogs are more than welcome at The Little Nell and when we checked in they gave Apollo a rawhide chew bone tied with a red ribbon. To this day I still have that red ribbon. The hotel staff told us if we were going out for dinner, a staff member could take Apollo out for a walk while we were gone. In addition, if we wanted someone to come in early the next morning he or she could take Apollo for a morning walk. As nice as the offer was there was no doubt we would still be taking my doggie for his walks; it was Apollo's trip as well as ours.

We asked if we could have a couple of buckets of ice delivered to our room, for Apollo of course. The Little Nell delivered the ice for Apollo, and champagne and strawberries for Joe, and all three of us sat out on the balcony enjoying a memorable afternoon…one big happy family.

After Joe and I came back from our dinner, Apollo woke up from his doggie nap and we were all ready for a nice long walk. Again, almost everyone we met along the way stopped to pet and ask about Apollo. After a longer than anticipated walk we went back to the hotel and thought we'd sit in front of the romantic fireplace in the main lobby and enjoy a quiet game of gin rummy with Apollo at our feet. Apollo lay sprawled out on the floor in front of the fireplace. From head to toe, he was almost six feet in length. He must have been quite a site, because as other hotel guests walked in and out almost everyone came over to ask what kind of dog he was, how much did he weigh, what his name was and of course, "Look at the size of those paws!" We had to laugh. We could almost anticipate the questions and it was the only game of gin rummy that three hours later, we still hadn't finished. Apollo, Joe and I enjoyed every minute.

We loved walking all around the gorgeous Colorado mountain town and the next morning hiked up the mountain right under the gondola. It was late October, and the last few aspen were losing their color and their leaves, it was cool, crisp and absolutely beautiful. We enjoyed the entire weekend; it was perfect. As we left we said to each other we must make the time to come back again.

As we were leaving the hotel that weekend, the hotel staff said, "Come back soon Apollo." Little did I know that would be Apollo's first and last trip to Aspen's The Little Nell.

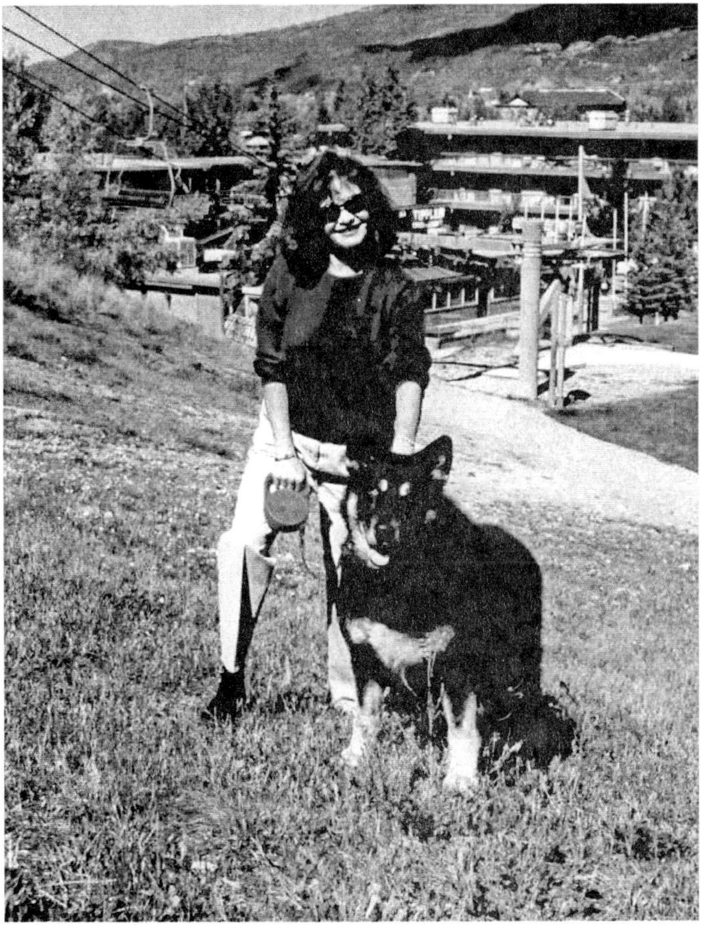

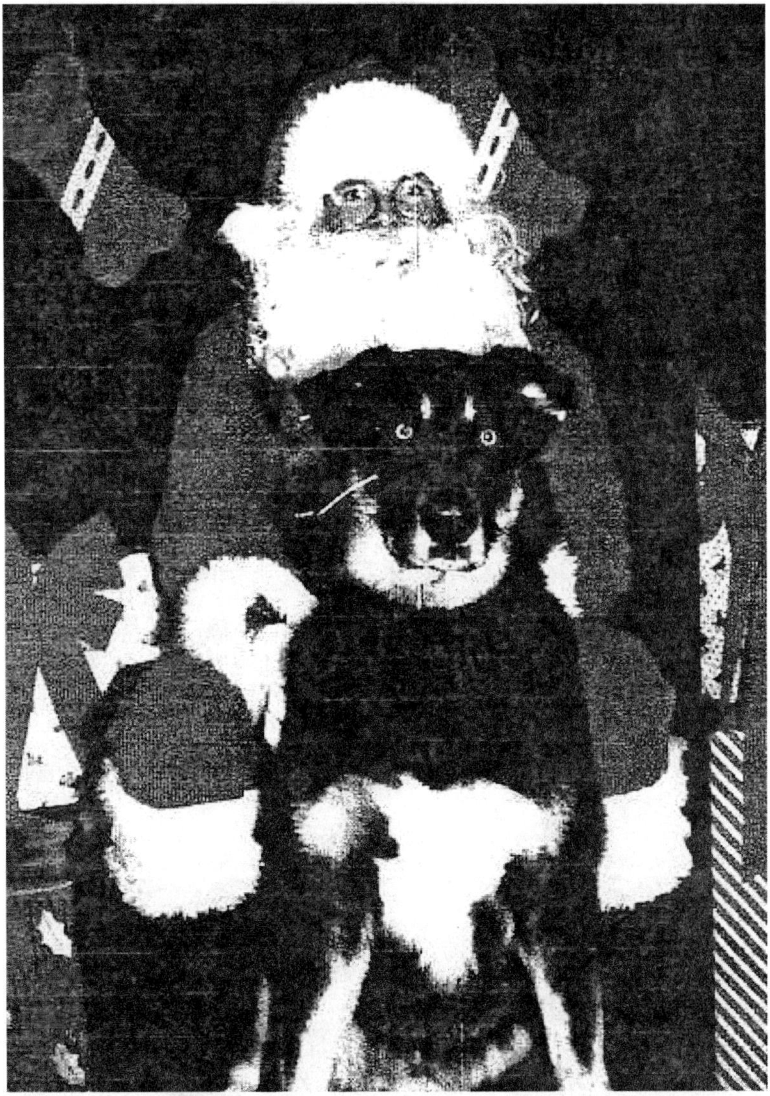

Our family drew names for a Christmas gift exchange. My dad drew my name and my dad kept phone calling me for my Christmas "wish list". I didn't really want to ask for anything so I turned things around and made it Apollo's "wish list" to my dad. Here is what Apollo wrote::

Dear Santa Claws

I have been a very very good dog this year due to the excellent training + care of my owner Debbie. So all I want for Christmas is a side of beef - and maybe some rawhide chews.

I would like a few things for my great owner — a fire extinguisher in case the Christmas trees catch on fire or she decides to try + cook. A 8-10 ft Aluminum ladder would be great so that she doesn't break her neck falling off that one she has. A salad shooter would be good since she's putting me on a diet Jan 1. And of course diamonds are a girls best friend (next to me of course) so earrings or an enhancer would be lovely.

By the way my cousins in Durango haven't told me what they want, so if you hear anything let me know. Just leave my side of beef next to my dish + I'll leave your Baileys + cookies on the coffee table.

Love, Apollo

Chapter 5

This Can't Be Happening to My Doggie

On Saturday morning December 14th, when we arrived with Apollo at Dr. Sara's office. We had the benefit of additional help and used a blanket underneath Apollo's stomach to help get him up, and give him some support. She wanted to watch Apollo walk to see if he could put any weight on his injured leg. Apollo yelped in pain. Apollo was a big, strong, tough dog and he rarely yelped, but he was crying out in pain. I fell to my knees and began to cry for him. This was my puppy, my best friend, and at that moment I couldn't do anything for him.

I hurt terribly knowing Apollo didn't understand what was going on. They took Apollo back to do x-rays and determine how bad the break was while Joe and I waited in another exam room. It was so hard. If I could have stayed with Apollo during this time it would have been so much easier for him. Dr. Sara came back in and showed us the x-rays. It was a bad break, almost a compound fracture and in a very awkward place. Dr. Sara said that even she couldn't set the bone and Apollo would need an orthopedic surgeon to re-set the bone. Joe asked if Apollo could recover at his age and size. Dr. Sara said that Apollo could indeed recover. She placed a call to the orthopedic surgeon and we began yet another long wait. Apollo was sedated with turbogesic and his leg was put in a heavy splint. Dr. Sara assured us that he didn't feel any pain, and explained that if a human took turbogesic prior to passing a kidney stone, they would feel absolutely nothing.

Apollo remained at Dr. Sara's office and I left without being able to give Apollo a hug because they were concerned if Apollo tried to get up or got excited, the broken bone would become a compound fracture. I left with a heavy heart and in tears. Apollo was in for some tough hours and there was nothing I could do. I felt like I was in as much pain as Apollo, emotionally at least.

The hardest part for me was knowing that Apollo couldn't possibly understand what was happening to him and that I was trying to do what I thought was best for him.

I thought that maybe Apollo would have surgery later that Saturday, but by the end of the day, Dr. Sara still hadn't heard back from the orthopedic surgeon's office. Dr. Sara took good care of Apollo, checking in on him frequently and making sure he was resting comfortably. Sunday came and went and there was still no call back from the orthopedic surgeons. I was becoming very anxious and upset. Apollo had never been confined to a kennel, and even though he was sedated I knew he wanted to be home.

Finally, on Monday, about midmorning, Dr. Sara called and let me know they had taken Apollo to the orthopedic surgeon's office. I was upset that I hadn't been with him for the trip to the orthopedic surgeon. I could have reassured him that everything would be alright and I know my hugs meant everything to Apollo. Monday afternoon I spoke with the orthopedic surgeon by phone. They had taken additional x-rays, put Apollo's leg back in a heavy splint and sedated him. I really wanted to see Apollo, but they continued to worry that he would get excited and possibly hurt himself even more so I reluctantly complied with their request not to see him.

Once I hung up the phone I sat down and cried. The orthopedic surgeon's office was waiting for the radiologist to read the x-rays. Late Monday afternoon I received a call telling me that because it was snowing the radiologist wouldn't be in until Tuesday. We had less than an inch of snow on the ground and I was very frustrated. I wanted Apollo's surgery done and I wanted him home; we had never been separated like this.

Finally, on Tuesday afternoon I received a call from the orthopedic surgeon. The radiologist had reviewed Apollo's x-rays and confirmed Apollo had a badly broken leg, and she determined it was a pathological fracture due to osteosarcoma-bone cancer. Those words hit me like a ton of bricks. BONE CANCER… how could this be possible? When I asked if they had done a bone biopsy I was told they hadn't. I just kept thinking this had to be a BIG, BIG MISTAKE! Apollo had gone from being a perfectly happy, healthy dog to a dog with a broken leg and bone cancer. This couldn't be true. There had to be a mistake. I strongly felt without a biopsy they couldn't diagnosis bone cancer but I was told the x-rays looked "typical" of bone cancer. My nightmare just kept getting worse! We set up an appointment for a consultation with the orthopedic surgeon to discuss our options.

I really wanted to see Apollo. I was tired of being told he was fine. I am sure being separated was every bit as hard on Apollo as it was on me. Joe and I once again sat in an exam room, this time at the orthopedic surgeon's office, waiting for our dog. When Apollo came in he looked at me with his big brown eyes as if to say, "Where have you been?" He seemed slightly drugged, but he was as happy to see me as I was to see him.

I sat on the floor and wrapped my arms around him, but it was a tearful reunion. His leg was heavily splinted and he had a hard time walking. The orthopedic surgeon sat down with us and told us they recommended amputating Apollo's leg and starting him on chemotherapy. We were told that this was the standard treatment for animals diagnosed with bone cancer in the limbs. We were told if we chose to do this treatment there was a forty to fifty percent chance that the cancer would not reoccur within a year.

I could not believe that even with the most radical, aggressive treatment, there was STILL a fifty to sixty percent chance that the cancer would reoccur within a year. We were also informed that limb salvage was not an option because that would only work if it were a front leg and the cancer was in Apollo's back leg.

If Apollo had not been such a big dog, the amputation might not have seemed so aggressive, but I wondered how in the world he would get around on three legs at 139 pounds. In addition, I had to consider his age, he was 9 and a half years old. It just didn't seem right to put a dog that old and that big through amputation and chemotherapy.

Intuitively, I knew that option was not the right treatment option for Apollo; I knew my dog well.

We asked what the prognosis would be if we chose to only repair the broken leg, and would the broken leg heal? The surgeon told us that if we did not choose the recommended treatment, Apollo would maybe live three to four months at best, and because bone cancer is painful, Apollo would live with a good deal of pain. Apollo's bone was capable of healing, but the cancer would spread very quickly.

I could not begin to describe the overwhelming feeling of helplessness I felt. There had to be another option in between the radical treatment recommended or putting Apollo to sleep.

I felt as if I were living a nightmare. What had started as a routine walk on a winter evening was now a dismal, hopeless picture of the future and the very imminent death of my best friend. I found the entire situation impossible to believe. Apollo had shown no signs whatsoever of being the slightest bit sick. He didn't have the sudden unexplained limp, supposedly the first symptom in the diagnosis of osteosarcoma in a dog. Apollo had been fine, excited as usual to go out for his evening walk. How could I just give up on my friend when he had nothing more than a broken leg, which could be fixed and heal?

My occupation was in the medical sales and I didn't want to put Apollo through chemotherapy. I had witnessed how people had suffered through chemotherapy and there wasn't any doubt in my mind I wasn't going to make Apollo go through that, even though I was told by the veterinary orthopedic doctor it was much easier on dogs than humans. Had I chosen chemotherapy for Apollo, either carboplatin or cisplatin, he most likely would have had to have gone through renal dialysis, a procedure to prevent kidney failure. I just couldn't do that to my best friend. Even though I was shown the additional x-rays and could see that where it was not broken the bone had a very mottled appearance, I wasn't ready to accept the diagnosis of bone cancer without a bone biopsy.

My other option was to put Apollo down, but as I sat on the floor scratching his chest, I looked at him and I didn't believe I could do that so suddenly. I also realized that no matter what I chose to do, my puppy dog was destined to die quickly. Apollo didn't seem ready to die, and I was not ready to give up on him over a broken bone. There had to be something else I could do.

Joe knew I was not about to give up exploring every imaginable option, so we kept pressing for more possible solutions. We asked about surgery to re-set the broken bone. We were re told that plates and screws could be used, just as they are in humans, but they would probably loosen in a few months and they didn't give much hope that Apollo would live comfortably, if at all, for more than three to four months without the chemotherapy. I refused to believe what I was hearing; from the looks of Apollo, he did not seem to be a dying dog!

Joe pressed on inquiring about surgery without plates and screws. The next alternative we were given was to use pins, some internal and some external, in order to provide support while the bone healed. Because much of the support would be external there wasn't the issue of screws loosening internally if the bone deteriorated. I asked about keeping Apollo's leg in the heavy splint. Keeping the splint dry was a big concern. We were approaching wintertime and snow in Denver, so that didn't seem like a good option.

The most important thing to me was Apollo's quality of life. Joe couldn't have said it better than when he told the orthopedic surgeon "it is more important for Deb to take Apollo home and spoil him every minute for whatever time he has left, than to extend his life if it is a miserable life." If Apollo's death was going to be sooner than I wanted or anticipated, whether it was three days or ninety days, they would at least be days I spoiled and loved Apollo.

I wanted to buy quality time with him. I wanted him home where he would be in his familiar surroundings and feel all the love he had felt his entire life. I needed more time to evaluate all my options for Apollo and I did not want to be rushed into making a decision that night.

So we took Apollo home with us. We were leaving with my slightly sedated puppy dog, and additional pain medication but WE WERE GOING HOME. I had a lot to think about but at least Apollo would be home, and we were going to be together again.

At the time Apollo broke his leg, he weighed 139 pounds. Because it was difficult for him to get up with the heavily splinted leg, we had to use a towel under his stomach to help get him up and into the car. Once we were home, it was even more difficult to get Apollo out of the car. Even when he didn't have a broken leg he would remain lying in the back seat of the car just because he wanted to. After all I was only the chauffeur; it was really always Apollo's car. When we would came home from a ride he would sometimes stay in the car for hours. I always propped open the door to ourhouse so he could come in whenever he wanted. Now, slightly sedated and splinted Apollo didn't want to move once we got home. We ended up bribing him with some of his favorite bacon treats, and between the two of us, Joe and I were finally able to get Apollo into the house. I didn't want him spending the entire night in the car because of his new "condition."

I put some big soft cushions from the couch on the floor in the family room, and I took Apollo his bowl of ice cubes and treats and set it beside him. My dog was home and nothing else mattered. I slept on the floor with my arms wrapped around Apollo scratching his chest. Because Apollo was still slightly sedated and groggy from the pain medication.

The following day brought more challenges, and he had a very difficult time getting up. We once again placed a big blanket under Apollo's stomach to provide him with support and help lift him so he could go out and walk around the back yard. His stiffly wrapped leg seemed to hinder Apollo from getting up with any ease. By the next day, Apollo was less drugged and managed, with great determination, to get up and go out, stepping off the deck into the back yard. He laid in the back yard as usual, rolling his face in the snow as he always did, he perked up and seemed happy for the first time in more than a week. That evening I sat in front of the fireplace at home with Apollo feeding him cold boiled shrimp. At that point, Apollo's cholesterol level was certainly not a concern. It was only his comfort and quality of life that was important. Apollo deserved to have anything he wanted to eat and I wanted to spoil him and make him happy, especially after what he had been through over the past few days.

I agonized for several days over what to do. I had intuitively known from the beginning of our ordeal that amputation and chemotherapy just did not seem to be the best option for Apollo. Chemotherapy was just too harsh; it would have killed good cells along with the cancer cells. And if had Apollo not been so big the amputation might have not been so bad, I just didn't feel he would be able to get up and around with only three legs. It was not acceptable to me that even with these drastic measures there was still a fifty to sixty percent chance that the cancer would return within one year.

My best friend knew what I was going through and gave me the name of a psychologist who had been through the amputation and chemotherapy with her golden retriever a few years prior. When I spoke with the psychologist she told me that her dog had lived for two years after she had been diagnosed, but that if she had to do it all over again she would not put a big dog through that course of treatment ever again. She told me that the chemotherapy made her dog sick and weak, maybe not to the same degree humans' experience, but still sick. My thought was, because dogs don't speak, it is difficult to determine how miserable they really feel. It is impossible for us to explain to our dog that the nausea, vomiting and sick feeling are only temporary and will help them and eventually make them feel better.

I didn't want Apollo's last months to be miserable for him. All I truly cared about was that for whatever was left of it, Apollo have a good life. It mattered more that he live a few months feeling near normal, going for his usual walks and eating his treats, than to live one to two more years and feeling sick the entire time.

I was trying to accept that Apollo and I didn't have much time left together. I had always thought he would live to be 15 to 16 years old. The realization that it would not be possible was devastating to me.

I chose to have Apollo's leg re-set using external pins and screws in hopes that Apollo's leg would heal so that he could at least go for walks again and have a few more months of attention and love. My biggest wish for Apollo was for him to be able to go for at least one more walk in the park. I wanted Apollo living the rest of his life spoiled, loved and feeling as good as he could. I didn't want the last days of his life to be in the hospital in unfamiliar surroundings and feeling miserable. It seemed to me the best option was to get the surgery over with as soon as possible and give Apollo the most normal and comfortable life he could possibly have for whatever time he had left at home.

I had been sleeping on the floor in the family room with Apollo since we brought him home. That night even though he had drifted off to sleep and seemed to be resting comfortably, tears were running down my face as I kept asking myself if I had made the right decision for Apollo. Was I short-changing him by not trying the chemotherapy? What about just the amputation? Many dogs live with just three legs. What if I helped him learn to walk with three legs? Apollo just didn't seem like he felt sick, except for the broken leg. I didn't think he seemed ready to give up and I didn't either. This was only the beginning of the many hard decisions I would have to make for Apollo over the next months. I just didn't know it at the time.

Chapter 6

Surgery... The Longest Wait

The next morning I called the orthopedic surgeon and scheduled Apollo's surgery for later that afternoon. My goal was to have Apollo get through surgery and come home as soon as possible. I was heavy-hearted and feeling helpless when I hung up the phone. How I dreaded taking Apollo back to the hospital again. In just a matter of days my best friend and I had gone from our annual Christmas tree shopping trip to facing Apollo's imminent death.

The years I had with Apollo were wonderful, and now, not knowing exactly how many minutes we had left, every minute with Apollo was a gift. I was so unprepared. I wondered how or if ever in my life I could really be ready to accept Apollo's death. I was not able to comprehend Apollo's impending death, just thinking about it was more than I could bare.

At that point I had to do everything I could to help Apollo. I wished I could have turned back the clock to the time when he was my little nine-week-old puppy. Our time together had just gone so quickly and I didn't want it to end.

During my lunch break that day I helped Apollo into the car for the ride back to the orthopedic surgeon's office for his surgery. It took 45 minutes of trial and error before I figured out a way to get Apollo from our family room to the car. We had to go up a few stairs, across the hardwood floor, out the door and down a few more stairs just to be able to get him into the car. And that was the easiest route! Apollo had lost weight and thenweighed about 130 pounds, and even though he was less sedated than a few days prior he just didn't have enough strength to hold up his body weight. I relied heavily on that large soft blanket under his stomach to help support some of his weight, but his heavily splinted leg dragged on the ground.

Several times we ended up sitting down to rest for a few minutes. It was hard for me and I hoped that it was not as hard for Apollo. Each time we sat down to rest Apollo put his chin on my shoulder and I scratched his chest and told him over and over, "You are going to be all right Apollo, we are going to get your leg fixed so that you can come home."

After several stops, we were close enough to the door for me to ask, "Apollo, do you want to go for a ride?" I hoped the familiar words and the jingling of my keys would inspire Apollo who usually bolted for the door and was ready to go every time he heard my car keys.

One of the most difficult things for me was to not cry, I knew that if I kept a calm soothing voice Apollo would not be afraid. With each step he took, I kept my voice steady and with each additional step I told him he was a "good dog."

Once we arrived at the orthopedic surgeon's office, I went in and asked for help getting Apollo out of the car. With two sets of hands he had a much easier time "hopping" on his three good legs. I gave Apollo a huge hug, told him he was a good dog he would be just fine, and told him I would be right back. As Apollo was lead back to the surgical area he looked back at me with his big brown eyes. By the time I got back to my car, tears ran uncontrollably down my face and I sat with my face buried in the steering wheel of the car.

Dr. Sara had told me that when I took Apollo home with his leg in a splint, I would know whether or not I should put him down. I still believed that if I had put Apollo down then without trying to do anything, and if his broken leg could heal, I would be giving up on him prematurely. I was convinced that if I could just get him through his surgery and get him home he could live a "normal" lifestyle happy as always, for as long as possible. As long as Apollo was interested in eating, sleeping and going for walks, life would be normal. Couch potato he was, I truly believed he would still be a happy dog.

Even though it was going to be hard for me, I didn't want to give up on Apollo without trying to help him first. I wanted to do everything, and I mean everything, for Apollo. Over our years together, Apollo had taken good care of me and I owed it to him to take extra good care him. He needed me more than ever.

I knew Apollo probably had cancer, but he didn't know and as long as I could keep a positive attitude, I felt he'd be none the wiser.

I received a call from the orthopedic surgeon's office late that Friday evening, Apollo's surgery had gone well and he was resting comfortably. They had inserted pins internally as well as externally. When I asked if they had done a biopsy, they told me they had performed a needle bone biopsy and the results would be available in a few days. I still had some hope, though slight, that the bone biopsy would turn up negative. I kept telling myself that Apollo had never been "normal" so why would that pattern change now? Even though his x-ray looked like typical osteosarcoma, knowing Apollo, it could have easily been something else. I prayed for a benign result.

A few days later, I learned the bone biopsy confirmed osteosarcoma; all I could do was cry.

Apollo was going to die sooner rather than later, and I could no longer deny it. I had wanted Apollo to be home by that Sunday. I called the orthopedic surgeon's office on Saturday to ask if I could see Apollo that day. The office staff told me it would be best if I could wait yet another day. I really didn't have a choice. I had no control in this situation.

CHAPTER 7

Life after Surgery

I was finally able to visit Apollo on Sunday, and on the way to the veterinary hospital, I stopped to get Apollo a cheeseburger. They told me they had been feeding him baby food since surgery. That fact alone was probably depressing to poor Apollo, so I thought a cheeseburger would cheer him up.

I sat with Apollo in the large dog run they had him in while he enjoyed his cheeseburger. Afterwards I placed hot packs on his leg, scratched his chest over and over and told him he would be home soon. He laid his head on my lap and looked up at me, and I knew all he wanted was to go home.

The orthopedic surgeon wanted to keep him yet another day. Monday came and went and they still wanted to keep Apollo another day. Each day I visited him and each time I left I felt a big hole in my heart and extreme emptiness. I wondered how in the world I would ever be able to deal with the day when Apollo didn't come home for good. Each day he spent at the veterinary hospital I felt like we were loosing ever so precious moments together. And worst of all I couldn't explain to Apollo what was happening. I felt so bad for him. He had never been kennelled and never been confined to a dog run. I knew this was hard on Apollo. On December 23, Apollo was finally released. Other than wishing the diagnosis of osteosarcoma was just a mistake, Apollo coming home was the only thing I wanted for Christmas. As Apollo and I drove away from the veterinary hospital, and holding back the tears as I said it, I promised him he would have a great Christmas. I was afraid it would be our last Christmas together.

That night, I brought several blankets and pillows down to the family room. I didn't want to leave him alone. We had already missed out on so much time together over the last couple of weeks. I didn't want to take a chance he would hurt himself trying to go upstairs on his own during the night.

I put Apollo's food and water dishes within easy reach so he wouldn't have to pull himself up from his stomach and drag himself across the room. He had developed a terrible rash from using his stomach to drag and pull himself up, and I wanted that rash and soreness to heal. I was determined to be there and help Apollo every step of the way. I wanted to make up for the burden of his broken leg. I was sure Apollo would be so much better after being home, despite the bleak picture that had been painted for us.

I left the Christmas tree lights on and snuggled up next to Apollo, scratching his chest. Soon he was breathing smoothly and was sound asleep. Thus began our new routine. We slept together on the family room floor and I made sure that anytime Apollo wanted to get up to move around I was there to help him. Christmas morning I awoke on the floor next to Apollo feeling very grateful. In just nine days he had gone from being perfectly normal to being diagnosed with osteosarcoma. Our choices were so limited, it seemed Apollo was doomed, but here we were, our first milestone. Even though I hadn't known it at the time, I had given Apollo a fighter name for a reason.

Apollo was amazing. He never seemed to be in pain once he was home, he almost immediately began to adjust for his broken leg, but of course Joe or I tried to always be there to ease some of the burden in getting up and outside. For Apollo, it was simply a new routine.

He had metal pins running from one side of his leg through to the other side and screws holding those pins in place, which meant I needed to clean the pins and screws several times a day because of the discharge of fluids. The pins and screws were fairly intricate and I had to clean them with swabs and warm water. It took about 20 to 30 minutes to clean them on both sides of Apollo's leg. The metal halo of pins and screws added weight to the leg. As I cleaned, the pins and screws he lay on his good side, and I positioned myself to use my legs as a prop for Apollo to rest his pinned leg on so he didn't tire the broken leg. He was stoic through the entire process.

The pins extended through the screws about a quarter inch top and bottom and had a tendency to catch on the fibers on the carpet. I thought that catching might cause some pain in the bone which was healing, so to eliminate that catching, I cut off the foot portion of all of my thick heavy slouch socks and doubled up a pair around the pins and screws at both the top and bottom. This not only eliminated the catching of the pins on the carpet, it kept Apollo from excessively licking at the pin and screw site, and it provided some absorbency for the discharge of the fluids. During this time, Denver experienced one of the worst arctic temperature spells in years. I knew that if I had holes drilled through my bones with metal pins entering one side and exiting the other the cold would be even worse, so I hoped the thick heavy socks would provide some warmth and protection from the cold.

Soon after, I made Apollo a fur "sleeve" to cover the pins. I used mink, rabbit or coyote fur and velcro to cover the four inch span from the top to bottom of the pin. After all, Apollo's natural fur had been shaved away for surgery and he didn't have any fur for protection or to keep that portion of his leg warm. I felt that if I could protect Apollo's leg from the cold arctic air we were experiencing, he would feel much more comfortable, and maybe even heal more quickly.

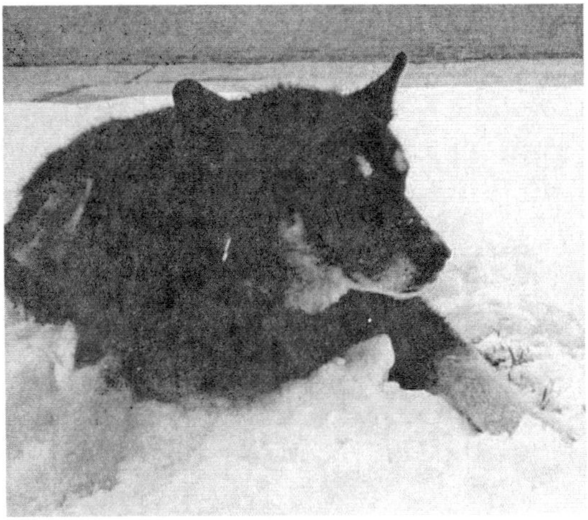

After close to two weeks in the veterinary hospital under the sedation of painkillers, confined in a very small area and being less mobile, Apollo was no longer housebroken. This was a situation I was not prepared for. I needed to find a way to know when Apollo had to go out and keep and eye on him if I wasn't within a few feet. I tied a small bell around Apollo's neck so that I could hear him when he got up from the floor and hear him if he went to the sliding glass door when he wanted to go outside.

I covered the family room floor with shower curtain liners and put comforters over the top of them to keep the carpet protected from any "accidents." I knew Apollo would have felt bad about accidents, so if I could clean up after him and make sure he always had fresh comforters to lay down on I thought he would feel better.

After a few days at home, Apollo was once again housebroken. I kept the fresh comforters on the floor, minus the shower curtain liners, to give him additional cushioning. Apollo seemed to be doing okay going outside when he needed to. I hoped this would be a major step for Apollo in getting back to a lifestyle as normal as possible.

I was concerned with Apollo's ability to get up off of the hardwood floors, especially his favorite spot right in front of the main entrance door of the house. The last thing Apollo needed was to be slip sliding on those floors again. I knew if he broke another bone that would be the end of his life. I went to the home improvement store and bought carpet floor runners with backing that gripped securely to the hardwood floors providing Apollo with a non-skid surface. I wanted him to be able to safely walk across the hardwood floors,whenever he needed or wanted. These runners remained on the floor for the remainder of Apollo's life, as ugly as they were; the point was to help Apollo and not to win an interior decorating contest. Those floor runners were a huge help in giving Apollo some sure footing and since most of the entries to the house were hardwood, with the exception of the back yard entry, I felt it was a necessity.

I slept on the floor with Apollo for the first four weeks he was home after his orthopedic surgery. I knew if he felt me close to him it would lessen the anxiety and discomfort he had from the broken bone and pins. Apollo usually laid on the side that didn't have the broken leg and I used pillows to prop up the leg with the pins and screws to relieve the stress on the healing bone. I thought elevating the leg slightly would keep any swelling minimized, and would make Apollo more comfortable. Not wanting to leave Apollo downstairs at night in case he needed anything, he was stuck with me as a "roomie."

Often, especially late at night, Apollo would want to go outside, not necessarily because he needed to go outside but to sit in front of the deck and just stare at the sky. He looked very much like the pictures of wolves looking up towards the sky. Apollo did this often through the last part of December and January, and did not seem to want to come back inside, which was unusual for him. It seemed like he was looking to the sky for answers, and once I realized this, I too would sit beside Apollo, my arms wrapped around his neck, looking to the sky for answers too; I was sure that together we would find them. I always brought out fur blankets or wraps and put them around Apollo to keep him and his broken leg warm. We were in this together and I was not going to leave him facing this fight and that uncertain time alone.

On many of these cold late nights together looking to the sky, I questioned what I was doing. I wondered if he was looking to the sky because he wanted everything to be over. Was he looking to the sky for hope? Was I doing the right thing for Apollo by not giving up on him and trying this surgery? Was I doing the right thing not doing the chemotherapy? Was I doing the right thing by not putting him to sleep now? I asked myself over and over again, "Am I doing the right thing for Apollo?"

I wanted Apollo to get well enough to go for another walk in the park to look for birds and rabbits. I wanted his last day to be happy- not miserable and in pain; a walk in the park, looking for the birds and trying to keep up with chasing rabbits. I found myself again hugging Apollow and telling him he would get better. He had such a strong personality and a great life so I truly felt he had a great will to live.

My dad often told me that Apollo had a better life than many children in this world and I realized that indeed might have been true.

The healing process on Apollo's broken bone was slow, difficult. Sometimes as Apollo and I were sitting outside in the cold nighttime air staring at the sky, I couldn't help but wonder if he had lost his spirit, his will to go on. But when we would go back inside the house and snuggle up in front of the fireplace, and as I would scratch his chest and give him a few treats he would look at me as if he really did understand and he wanted to go on.

Every night, Apollo waged his tail and licked my face before falling asleep. He seemed happy to be home. I just wanted him to feel better soon and have some happy walks before it was time to say our final goodbye. I knew we had just a little time, but I hoped and prayed that the time would be on Apollo's side. I wished that Apollo knew he would feel better soon, and that we could once again go for our normal walk in the park together. I was determined to make it happen for Apollo.

A few days later, Denver once again experienced an unusual and severe cold spell in January with temperatures below zero degrees for several days in

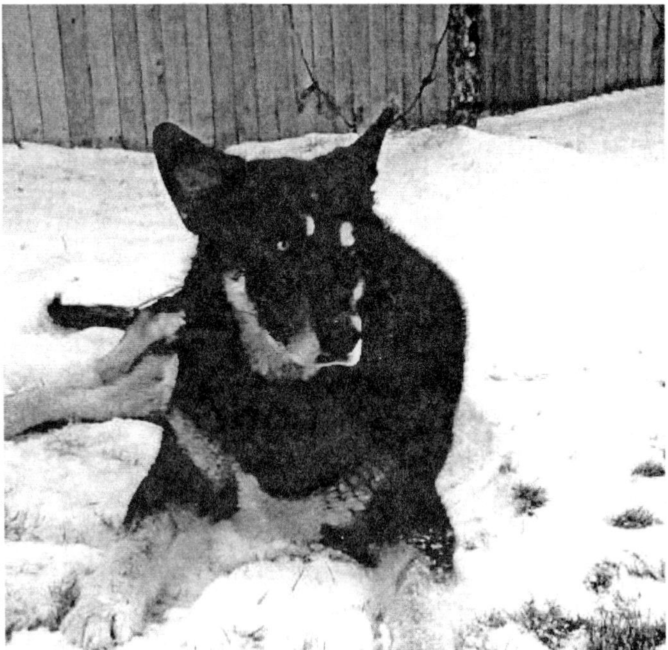

a row. I sensed that Apollo was feeling more pain after he'd been outdoors. So, after letting him back inside I would give him a warm bowl of chicken or beef noodle soup. After he finished the soup he would lay on his side and I would wrap his broken leg with a moist heating pad to warm and relax his muscles, then remove the moist heat pack and wrap his leg in a small fur blanket. Soon afterward, he would be sound asleep looking comfortable.

I moved my office to a makeshift space in the family room, cordless phones took on a whole new meaning, the giant coffee table became my desk and Apollo and I "officed" together. His office space just happened to be the prime space in front of the fireplace, and he didn't have to worry about paying rent. We would get through this cold spell together. Knowing it was literally "bone-chilling" to Apollo, I was determined to keep him as comfortable as possible.

I noticed that after coming in from the cold Apollo would often pull his broken leg up towards his chest; in physical therapy, it is known as "guarding." Guarding can often lead to muscle spasms and pain because the muscles remain in a contracted state for extended periods of time. I began to massage Apollo's leg, hip area above and below the pins and into the area around his paws. Each time I did this, Apollo would stop guarding and I could feel his muscles relax. Once he relaxed, he didn't have any more muscle spasms, and soon afterward he started getting up without my help and moving to other places in the family room. I was more encouraged each time Apollo got up on his own and walked to another place in the room. I felt like it was another milestone. Apollo appeared to be gaining more strength and courage, and I felt even more strongly that Apollo wanted to live. I had to give him that chance. I couldn't quit. Apollo didn't want to quit, I was very sure of that. I told myself I just needed to be patient until his broken bone healed.

Some days were very good and some days were very bad. It was a combination of great ups, and earth-shattering downs. One of those earth-shattering downs came just a few weeks after it appeared Apollo was starting to heal. I took him to the orthopedic surgeon's for his post-surgery check-up; Apollo's leg had suddenly become very swollen.

The orthopedic surgeon's staff took new x-rays while I waited in yet another exam room for Apollo to come back and be with me. I was fed up with us being separated. The orthopedic surgeon interpreted the x-ray's and told me that from the x-rays the tumor appeared to be very aggressive, and that in most cases when they saw these types of x-rays the dog didn't live much longer.

How could this be happening?

Apollo seemed to be feeling so much better. He was starting to get up and walk around, I was finally beginning to have some hope that we would have more time together, and that Apollo would be able to go for another walk in the park. How could everything, once again, seem to be falling apart? I really had believed that we could make it at least another six months, and now I was hearing this devastating news from his veterinarians? Being told he probably only had a couple more weeks at best, how could I possibly be ready to tell my best friend goodbye?

I thought we were making some progress.

I had promised him another walk in the park!

I held back the tears as we drove home from the orthopedic surgeon, I felt I had to keep a positive attitude for Apollo.

When we arrived home I gave him his warm soup and he laid down in front of his new favorite spot in front of the fireplace and fell asleep. Apollo seemed just fine. He didn't notice his leg was swelling and he also didn't seem to be in any pain, what was I supposed to do for him now? I asked myself if I was making Apollo suffer in any way, and I could not answer my own question.

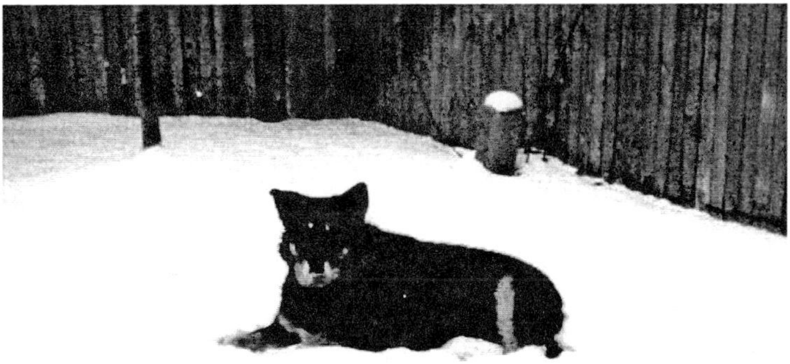

I went upstairs to my room, buried my head in the pillows and cried and cried. I cried so hard I could hardly breathe. I just couldn't imagine being without my best friend. We had been through so much together for these almost ten years. I had awoken every day with his chin on my pillow looking at me and ready to go for his walk. There wasn't a night that we were home together that I didn't fix him his bowl of ice cubes and treats and place them at the foot of the bed, hugging him and telling him what a good dog he was.

How could I say goodbye? Could I ever accept saying goodbye?

I wondered how my best friend, so gentle, so treasured and so loved could be slipping away right before my very eyes. I didn't have any answers. Apollo had been just fine until that awful Friday night after his routine nightly walk. I could not say goodbye. I had to do more, but what? I was running out of time and options, yet what else could I do? There had to be something else I could do for Apollo, the question was what?

A few days later as Apollo lay in my office I noticed his leg was bleeding. I made a call to the orthopedic surgeon's office and the resulting answer brought more bad news.

They said the bleeding was probably a sign that the tumor was growing. Again I was told Apollo probably didn't have much time to live.

As I lie awake each night listening for Apollo's bell, ready to help him out or just move about, I kept asking myself if there was anything more I could do. I just couldn't accept being so totally helpless.

Apollo didn't seem ready to lay down and die and I couldn't let him. I had promised him, at the very least, one good last walk in the park, so it was time to step up the assistance in Apollo's fight.

Chapter 8

New Hope and Help for Apollo

As I was thinking about Apollo's situation late one night I asked myself what more could I do for Apollo? When the orthopedic surgeon confirmed the biopsy on Apollo's leg I was told that bone cancer was extremely painful. I recalled an article I had saved several years before from a local newspaper.

The article was about a Colorado veterinarian who performed acupuncture on dogs with hip dysplasia to help with movement and control pain. I had saved that particular newspaper article because Apollo's puppy veterinarian, and several of my friends with dogs had all told me that because of Apollo's breeding and size he would probably end up with hip dysplasia as an older dog.

I had saved that newspaper article for a reason. In the middle of the night I tiptoed down to the basement to search for that article and the name of the veterinarian.

If acupuncture could control the pain associated with hip dysplasia, I thought there was a possibility it might also control the pain associated with the bone cancer. I searched several hours that night for the newspaper article and finally found it.

I had such a sense of hope and relief that maybe, just maybe, I could finally do something to help Apollo.

I immediately called the veterinarian's office and made an acupuncture treatment appointment. For the first time in many, many weeks I had hope that maybe there would be help. For the first time that night I didn't cry myself to sleep. I could at last do something to take care of him.

On our way to Aspen Park Veterinary Hospital, I realized what a long drive it was 37 miles one way from our house. I hoped it would be worth it. I didn't mind the drive as long as the acupuncture treatments would help Apollo. I kept telling him over and over he would feel better soon because he was going to get some help.

We checked into a busy veterinary office and I filled out all of the required new patient paperwork. The office staff asked if, in addition to the acupuncture, I was interested in trying everything I could do for Apollo. *Of course I was interested in hearing more about any possible options which would benefit Apollo!*

At that first appointment I met "Doc," as he is affectionately known. Doc reviewed all of Apollo's x-rays, laboratory reports and notes from the other veterinarians. Doc performed a thorough exam on Apollo before he began an acupuncture treatment. While Apollo received the acupuncture, Doc suggested giving Apollo daily doses of vitamin C - a publicly well-known anti-oxidant which might also boost his immune system in fighting the cancer. Doc also suggested Feverfew, a natural herbal supplement which is also a well-known pain reliever. I preferred that to a heavy dose of narcotics, which I had been told previously Apollo would probably need.

I was relieved to have the acupuncture as another pain management option available to Apollo. Doc also told me that "cancer is a great teacher." I was not happy about that "lesson" having to be learned through and at my best friend's expense. I was hoping that between the acupuncture and feverfew, the combination would be successful in keeping Apollo comfortable because I really did not want Apollo drugged on heavy narcotics; after all everything I was doing was about preserving his quality of life. If he was constantly drugged, what would be the point? This journey was about Apollo, not about me. I drove home from Aspen Park Veterinary Hospital and for the first time in six weeks, I felt there was at last some hope. Apollo rode home with his head sticking out the window enjoying the fresh winter air.

One of the most helpful things Doc suggested for Apollo was the "walk-about." The best way I can describe it is an apparatus/harness with handles on both sides that fits around the dog to assist getting up and around; basically a lift for Apollo. The walk-about harness was so much better than the blanket under his stomach, and it quickly helped to eliminate the rash on Apollo's stomach. Apollo's walk-about became his new fourth leg. He never knew I had him by the handles to help him about on his reengineered fourth leg. This was another victory for Apollo, maybe our walk in the park would be also just around the corner.

I had been doing extensive research on shark cartilage. According to the research, there was a theory that shark cartilage had an angiogenic effect on tumors. There was evidence that eliminating the source of nourishment to the tumor could result in shrinking the tumor and starving the tumor by stopping the blood supply, which made sense. I searched for high-quality shark cartilage, ordered some and began giving it to Apollo. I knew it could not hurt him, and even if it did not shrink the tumor it might help the joints and bones that had been taking up the slack for Apollo's broken leg.

Apollo also began a regimen of vitamins, colloidal minerals and antioxidants. Because it was winter and cold outside, I broke open the capsules of shark cartilage, vitamins and antioxidants into Apollo's warm soup. I added the colloidal minerals to his regular drinking water. Three or four times a day I would make this healthy doggie soup and warm it for him when he came in from outside. It was easy to find a lot of variations in chicken and beef soups to mix in all of the supplements and it was good to see Apollo enjoy the treat. I felt that getting Apollo warmed up quickly when he came in from the outside would help ease any possible pain. Once again Apollo had me trained and I was now his "personal chef."

I continued applying the moist heating pad on Apollo's broken leg when he came back in from outdoors. Every morning, lunch break and evening I massaged all of Apollo's legs. Since he was putting more pressure on his healthy legs, I wanted to prevent those legs from feeling sore from the added pressure and weight they were supporting due to the broken leg. I also continued gently moving his pinned leg, similar to what is done in physical therapy on humans. As Apollo lay on his side I would move the broken leg back and forth very slowly and then massage it until I felt it relax. I had done some research on muscles and memory and learned that if muscles are not used for extended periods of time, in addition to atrophy the muscles would lose memory, they could forget how to move normally.

I was not trained to do physical therapy, I just used what I thought was common sense and judged Apollo's reaction in order to determine if what I was doing was helpful in making Apollo feel better. When I gently moved and massaged Apollo's pinned broken leg, his reaction was very similar to when I would scratch his chest, so I took it as a good sign when I felt his entire body and muscles relax. Joe and I often watched Apollo as he lay sleeping and he moved the broken leg back and forth as if he were dreaming he was chasing rabbits. I thought Apollo must be feeling a little better, and I hoped that someday he would once again be able to chase rabbits without any help from me.

Five to six weeks after beginning the combinations of all of the treatments, I began to notice that Apollo seemed to be feeling much, much better. It was a huge relief. He was getting up and moving around much more often without any of my help. Despite the bleak prognosis from the orthopedic surgeons, I had hoped that Apollo's leg would heal and that he would feel good for the remainder of the time he had left. I still wanted Apollo to be able to go for that one last walk in the park on his own.

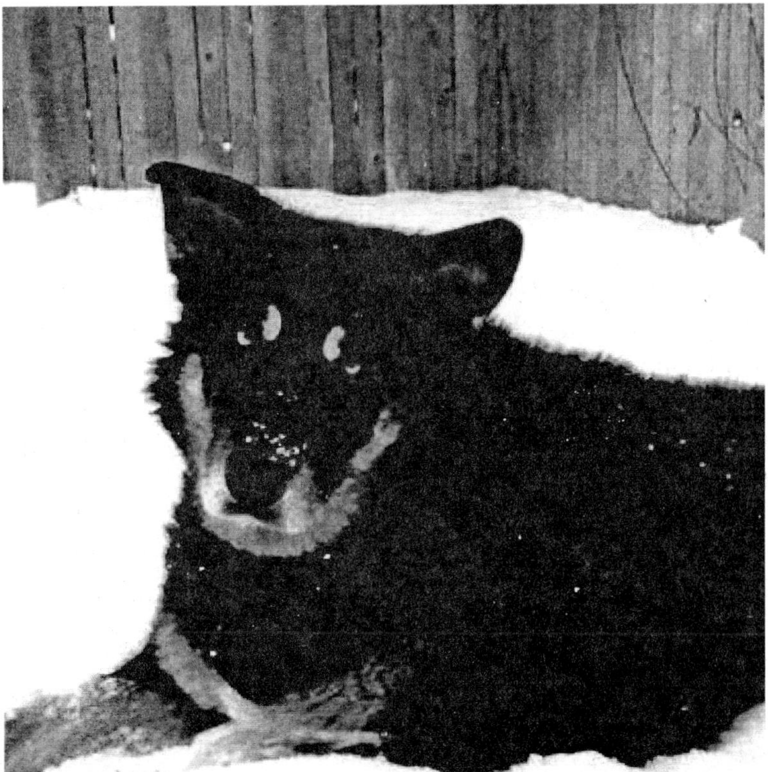

Chapter 9

A Resort Dog Once More

Apollo was feeling so well that when my brother and sister-in-law invited us to join them in Telluride, we decided to take the trip with Apollo. Apollo was used to traveling, so the seven and a half hour drive was not a problem for him. We stayed at The Peaks Resort and just like The Little Nell, The Peaks also welcomed dogs.

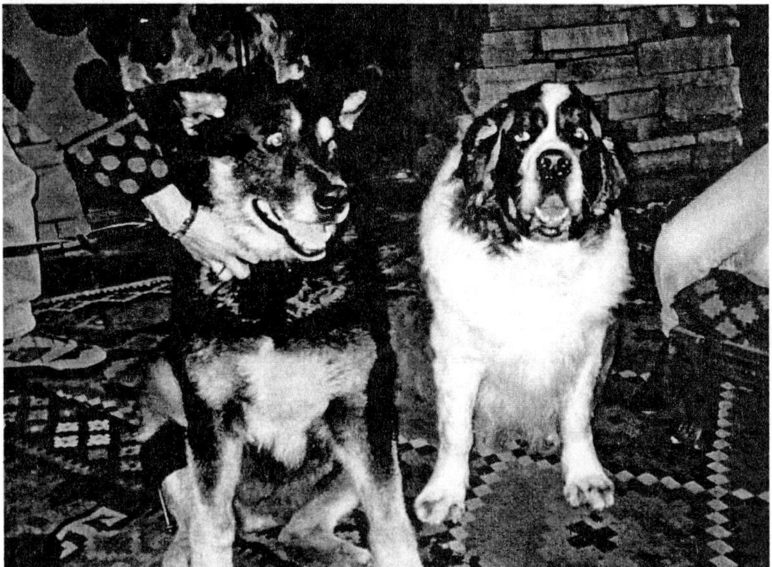

When Joe, my brother and sister-in-law skied, Apollo and I walked around in the snow. There was a lot of snow! I helped Apollo walk with the walk-about because I didn't want him to have the extra weight of the snow on his pinned leg. I treasured the many short walks Apollo and I took together. After our walks, we'd go back to the room and clean his pins as usual, massage his legs and warm him up.

Apollo would then be ready for his nap. Once again, he was a big hit at the resort. One afternoon we sat in front of the big roaring fireplace in the lobby and Apollo met a beautiful St. Bernard. Apollo was at least as big as the St. Bernard.

Other than the slouch socks covering Apollo's pins he looked and acted like a normal healthy dog. He rolled his face in the snow on our walks, and I knew he was a happy dog. For the first time I did not question the decisions I had made in Apollo's treatment.

The month was February and according to the statistics Apollo should have been dead, instead he enjoyed the snow and being a "spa" dog for the weekend. Apollo enjoyed his last trip to a Colorado mountain resort. He had made it past another milestone; he was living pain-free and moving about when he was supposed to be dead. Apollo was beating the odds, I was grateful for each and every minute I had with him and even happier that he was happy and pain-free. It almost seemed too good to be true.

Chapter 10

A Few Bumps in the Road

Apollo's broken bone was healing, but we did go through times when I could tell he wasn't feeling well. Each time we would hit a "bump" I felt a big lump in my throat, not knowing if this was going to be "the end." Apollo would feel bad for one or two days and then he would get better and feel good again. A long as Apollo could bounce back, then so could I. He showed an interest in doing all of the things dogs do: eat, nap and excitedly greet me when I came home from work. I gladly did anything for my best friend, as long as he felt good we would go on.

One of the brightest moments I remember in Apollo's recovery was in March. It was spring break and Joe's son was visiting us. Three and a half months after he had been diagnosed with bone cancer, Joe, his son and I took Apollo for his first nice long walk! We used the walk-about for support. Joe held up one side and I held the other, and Apollo took off like he was running in a race, he really took Joe and I for a run! It was hard to keep up with him. I could have fallen face first to the ground and it would have not mattered to me, Apollo was going for a walk! I promised Apollo another walk in the park and I had never broken any promises I made to him. I was now 100 percent sure Apollo would walk in the park again.

We walked a block and a half and Apollo would have kept walking, but we didn't want him to overdo it end up sore. Even though Apollo needed our help, he wanted to walk! For the first time in more than four months, tears of happiness instead of anguish ran down my face.

Apollo was getting better. So as we sat in the front yard, I took Apollo's leash off and for the first time since the horse playing incident he was really off leash. Sadly though I knew that if he did get up to try and chase a rabbit he could not get very far by himself.

Thus began a new chapter in Apollo's life. After our walks I would let him off his leash and he would lie in the middle of the front yard happy to observe everything going on around us. There were a few times he caught sight of a rabbit and tried and chase it. That was a GREAT sign! I had to laugh, Apollo would lay off leash and stay in the front yard, freedom from the leash at last, and when other dogs walked by Apollo would perk up his ears and watch, content to just observe. Apollo had finally learned a down stay without a leash! Of course those down stays were on his terms, some things hadn't changed and Apollo did what he wanted to do, when he wanted to do it.

From March to June, Apollo had a couple of "sick" days. Some weeks we made trips to Aspen Park two or three times to do whatever it took to get Apollo feeling better again. Apollo and I shared many morning sunrises together on our way to those 7:30 a.m. appointments. Our trips provided me with the opportunity to enjoy the quietness and appreciate the beautiful sunrises, which I had really never stopped to appreciate before.

Several times during the course of that spring and summer Apollo developed slight infections. I thought that was understandable, after all his body was trying to fight a big infection - CANCER. Doc usually gave Apollo an injection of antiobiotics and sometimes in addition oral antibiotic's, sometimes I fretted over doing too much for Apollo and once again questioned what I was doing, hiding oral antibiotic's in soft cheese seemed sneaky to me. However when I mentioned my concern to Doc he said, "You are saving your dog's life and preserving his quality of life."

After one of our early sunrise trips to Aspen Park, I came home and was anxious to hurry and get to work but Apollo had a different idea. He walked around the front yard for a while, and at my very favorite rose bush he literally stopped and sniffed the roses. I looked at him in amazement. It had been so many months since I had taken the time to enjoy any of my roses! I sat down for a little while watching Apollo and I realized that maybe life is too short. My best friend was dying and he was "telling" me to stop and smell the roses. That night after our walk, I cut several roses from that rose bush, put them in a vase and after they wilted and died I dried them. To this day, I still have the dried rose petals in my office. They are a reminder from Apollo to take a few minutes to stop and smell the roses.

Chapter 11

Oh what a relief! Once again who is walking whoM?

On Sunday, Father's Day, we were having a very big "bump" with Apollo. His broken leg had begun to swell terribly. It looked like a small balloon had been inserted between the pins, and the pins kept getting tighter and tighter. We looked at each other and Apollo helplessly, his poor leg looked like the water balloon was ready to burst.

We talked about, "What if this was it?" Apollo had been doing so well and now this huge mass seemed to be growing on his leg. Was the cancer beginning to overcome Apollo? We called Doc and in

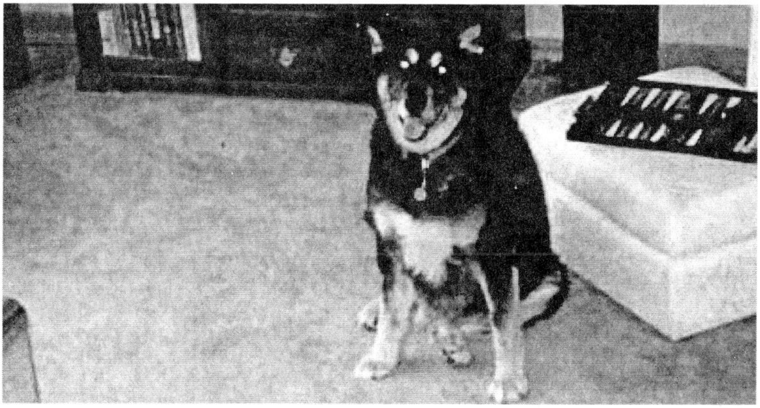

his calm manner he assured us he would see Apollo the next morning. We snuggled up on the floor with Apollo, not knowing if Apollo would even be there with us the next night. It was impossible to even sleep that night, Apollo didn't seem to be in any pain, but his leg looked awful.

The next morning brought another sunrise drive to Aspen Park. Doc loosened the external pins, which Apollo had since his orthopedic surgery more than six month's prior, to give Apollo more room. There was no doubt that there was a huge mass growing on Apollo's leg, yet even when Doc or I touched it or put pressure on it Apollo did not seem to be in pain. The next few weeks became more difficult, as the external mass grew larger and larger; I was worried that that cancer was taking over. Doc took chest x-rays of Apollo and his lungs were clear, so the cancer had not metastasized to his lungs, which is where the cancer usually spreads first. At least the cancer didn't appear to be spreading internally. At least there was some good news.

After another couple of weeks the mass began to bleed, not a whole lot, however it was enough to need bandages... I was hoping and I was praying that the external mass would shrink and stop bleeding.

Amazingly, Apollo did not even notice the huge mass. He was able to take the big step off the back yard deck and walk by himself around the house and yard. As long as Apollo seemed to feel fine, I couldn't give up and put him down, he was just not ready to stop fighting and neither was I.

When we asked Apollo if he wanted to go for a walk he still got excited and went to the front door just waiting for us. Using the walk about, we were still able to take Apollo for his walks - he didn't seem to notice that we were "helping" and he still pulled us. He did have a limp, however it just didn't seem to bother him, even though it continued to bleed and grow.

I began changing Apollo's bandages three or four times a day, it was an absolute necessity. By the beginning of July, the space between Apollo's leg and the external pins was gone - my heart sank. The leg and the mass were very swollen. On an early Saturday morning, Doc removed all of the external pins from Apollo's leg. The x-rays of the leg showed the bones in the leg had healed, the question was whether or not the leg was strong enough to support Apollo's weight, he weighed about 120 pounds now.

I knew that if he re-broke his leg that would be the end of our time together. I continued to do everything I could possibly do to keep from amputating Apollo's leg and I wondered if I had pushed him too far. What was I doing for or to my dog?

It was difficult to sleep at night even as I heard Apollo with his normal breathing as I lay awake. Was I pushing too hard or was I not trying hard enough? I wrestled with that question for endless nights. I wondered what Apollo would do if he were in my place, continue on or say goodbye? I believed he would have stood by my side and continued to do everything he could.

Once again, Apollo lead me in the direction I thought he'd have gone (if he were in my position), after all he trained me very well to do just as he wanted from the time he was a puppy.

We celebrated the Fourth of July at home, watching fireworks from the front yard. Of course, as usual, Apollo seemed to enjoy the show. Apollo had always gone to fireworks shows and liked them-unusual for many dogs - but then again, Apollo was never "usual." It was, however, a "cautious" celebration even knowing that Apollo was beating the odds, he was now in the seventh month after being diagnosed with his bone cancer, almost twice as long as he had been expected to live without doing chemotherapy. He still had a great spirit, his appetite was good, he still wanted to go for walks and he did not act like a dying dog or a dog that was ready to die. However, the mass continued to bleed and grow and I began to worry even more.

One of the other big challenges was to keep Apollo from chewing through his bandages. I used a lot of bitter apple on the vet wrap to try and keep Apollo from chewing them. Several times I came home from work to find Apollo having chewed through the bandages and the bloody mass and he was bleeding all over the carpet. I had switched from just vet wrap on the outside of the bandages to duct tape on top of the vet wrap, which was much harder for Apollo to chew through. That was a huge help. The duct tape might not have tasted very good to Apollo, another deterrent and he really began to chew less on his bandages.

However, the mass started to bleed so much that I had to change the bandages outside our house And I changed from using the usual type first aid bandages to using feminine sanitary pads as bandages to stop the bleeding. Sometimes as I was changing the bandages blood would shoot out of the mass. Through all of this, Apollo STILL didn't seem to feel any pain, and he was quite used to lying on his side when I propped up his leg to change the bandages.

On many, many occasions I wondered, "What am I doing to my dog?" However, Apollo seemed fine, if you had not seen the huge bulky bandages on his leg, he appeared to be a normal dog. I just couldn't imagine putting him down just because the mass was a bloody mess. I just wanted to do the right thing for Apollo, and it did not seem like Apollo was ready to go.

The hardest thing I did was leave Apollo for a few days in August. Joe had promised his mom and stepdad a visit from us. I asked Doc if I could leave him with his practice. He needed so much care and I knew I would be leaving Apollo in great hands with Doc and his staff. I knew he would have the very best care and attention. Doc, of course agreed to keep Apollo, however, Doc said that Apollo might make his permanent exit while I was gone. I had to be willing to accept that whatever happened. I didn't have any control over it.

With a huge lump in my throat and tears in my eyes I hugged Apollo as I left him. I promised him I would be back soon. The tears would not stop as I left. While I was gone, I called Doc's office every day to check on Apollo, and get a progress report, fortunately, each day I hung up the phone with a sigh of relief. Apollo was doing fine. When we arrived back in Denver, I immediately went to pick Apollo up from Aspen Park. He easily got up. He was very excited to see me and he looked great! The mass had reduced considerably. This was a sign Apollo was definitely not ready to make his final exit. My dog wanted to keep going on with me.

Apollo did well for another few weeks, but then the mass began to bleed even more profusely and grow again. It seemed there was truly a battle between Apollo and his leg. I began to get up during the night to change Apollo's blood-soaked bandages. We would go out onto our deck, change the bandages and then go back upstairs to sleep. Apollo would easily fall asleep, but I could not. I felt like our options were running out and yet I felt as if I chose to let Apollo go, I would be giving in because of me having to do some messy work.

Apollo bled all over the car and all over the carpet in the house and it was not easy to keep him from bleeding through his bandages. One Saturday morning, he bled very badly and I was out of bandages. So I put big bath towels in the back seat of the car and went through the pharmacy drive-thru. I explained our situation and asked if they could please get me the bandages for Apollo's leg. Even though it wasn't a prescription, they did help Apollo and brought the bandages to the window. To this day I am extremely grateful. I did everything possible for Apollo to keep his leg, it gave him some balance and I thought that was helpful to him. Everything I chose to do was all about Apollo and what was best for him. I believed he'd beat the odds and I thought he could continue to do so.

Finally, by the first of September, I had to admit that Apollo's leg was not ever going to heal, I felt like I had tried everything. I was concerned with Apollo losing so much blood. I worried about him becoming weak and anemic, so I began giving him beef liver, that was a treat for him.

On one of our visits to Doc, I had to ask if it was time for me to do what I had avoided for almost ten months and remove his leg. Apollo had lost a lot of weight. Doc, once again did x-rays to determine if the cancer had spread to other internal organs. The x-ray results showed the cancer had not spread to his lungs or any other major organs. Other than that leg, Apollo seemed fine, I once again had to make a very hard decision for him.

Chapter 12

Considerations in Removing Apollo's Leg

It was a terrible struggle to even consider the possibility of removing Apollo's leg. For months I had done everything possible for him to keep it, because I thought that was the right thing for him. Now it was becoming very clear to me that I really had no choice, it was either Apollo or his leg. He could no longer live with the leg like it was, and finally, I accepted it would never get better.

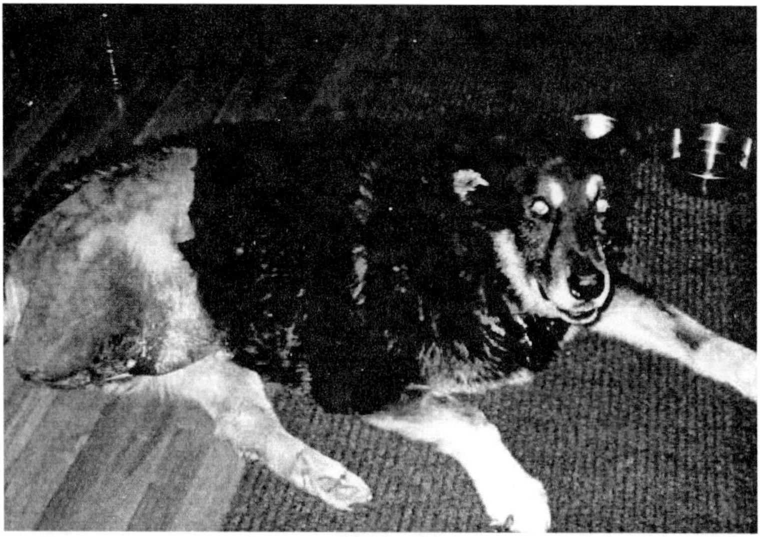

However, his circumstances had changed so much, since he initially broke his leg. Now it was not removing a leg that was broken, it was a leg that was the only sign Apollo was "sick," and keeping the leg was only causing terrible bleeding for Apollo. I felt he needed his strength to continue to try and fight the cancer.

I kept reminding myself that he was now down to 119 pounds, a healthier weight for him. That was a significantly less amount of weight for the other three legs to support. Apollo also had about nine months to adjust to relying on only three legs and really not using that fourth leg too much. He basically limped on it. Finally, Apollo still showed an interest in doing what dogs do best: sleep, eat, go for walks and get a lot of love and attention from their owner.

Apollo had really always been pretty much a "couch potato" dog, if he had been a working dog I would have made different choices. And from the x-rays, his lungs, liver, spleen and pancreas all looked tumor free. Removing Apollo's leg really seemed to be the only choice left for me to make for him.

He just didn't seem ready to say our final goodbye and his leg was the only part of his body which did not seem to be cooperating with him. After a lot of tears and consideration I decided to amputate Apollo's leg that weekend, it was Labor Day weekend and I knew I would have one extra day to take good care of him.

Apollo and I drove to Aspen Park at about noon and as we made the drive Apollo had his head out the window as usual, seeming to enjoy the fresh air,

I had tears welling in my eyes. Was I betraying my best friend or was I helping him? I prayed that my decision would indeed help him. Doc also told me before beginning the surgery that Apollo might not wake up from surgery. I had to understand that was once again something I didn't have any control over.

Doc always let all of his patients stay with their pets during their exams and acupuncture treatments. I *never* had to wait in the lobby or another exam room. I was fortunate to always be at Apollo's side to comfort him. Doc then also took us to an exam room together and to read Apollo's radiograph's. On the viewer right in front of me, he explained the interpretation. I went outside, waited nervously and prayed and looked at the mountains and the aspen trees changing their color. Less than a year ago, Apollo had been walking under a gondola in Aspen, what seemed unimaginable then was a harsh reality now.

Doc's staff constantly updated me as the surgery progressed, Apollo was hanging in there. I just didn't want to lose him. It was now up to Apollo to wake up. I hoped that I had chosen the right option for my little dog. I had to live with my choice no matter what the outcome. Less than an hour later, I was able to go back into the recovery unit after Apollo was closed and sutured. Doc had performed the entire surgery in about an hour. And the staff told me that after Doc stapled Apollo's surgical site, Apollo began to stir. He was starting to wake up! What a good sign; Apollo was continuing to fight his battle-he wanted to live!

Doc and his assistants picked Apollo up from the surgical table and put him in the recovery suite on the floor on a blanket which had Charlie Brown characters and that read, " It's Good To Have A Friend." I was re-united with him and sat down next to him scratching his chest and petting his head. I just wanted him to know I was still there with him.

At about 3:30 p.m., Apollo began to really wake up, he tried lifting his head and then his body. Doc had remained with Apollo and me through his recovery and as Apollo began to get up.

Doc said, "That dog is really amazing!" Doc in all of his wisdom knew Apollo wanted to continue on. Apollo was definitely a fighter. He told me to wait with Apollo for about another hour and then he would check back on Apollo and if everything looked good, we could probably go home.

The words, "You could probably go home." signified yet another victory for Apollo. He just had his leg amputated just a couple of hours prior. I expected to re-live Apollo's first surgery. Yet, Apollo and I left Doc's office about 4:30 p.m. that same day. We were home by 5:30 p.m., just hours after removing Apollo's leg. Apollo did not have to stay for days in the hospital as he did his first surgery. Joe arrived home from work a little later and with assistance from both Joe and I, we enticed Apollo out of the car with some freshly cooked bacon and went to the back yard.

Apollo was still a little groggy and went to sleep on the deck. I felt a huge relief and in my heart I felt I had done the right thing for Apollo by removing his leg. We stayed in the back yard on the deck with

Apollo until late into the night as he lay sleeping on the deck. There would not have to be any bandage changing that night for Apollo, he could sleep without that mess interrupting him for the first time in months. I went upstairs grabbed a pillow and blanket, put everything up on the outdoor lounge chair and slept on the deck, I wanted to make sure I was there for Apollo when he woke up the next morning. I did not want him to be alone, he had chosen to keep on going and I wanted to be there to thank him.

Chapter 13

A New Day & What A Relief!

On Saturday morning, Apollo woke up and began to walk around the back yard as if nothing happened! He walked as well as if he had all four legs! I was totally astounded! He did not seem to be groggy; he didn't have extra weight or a bloody mass holding him back. Of course, Apollo did not walk as if he knew he had his leg removed. I would have never guessed he was missing a leg. He was the most mobile I had seen him in the last ten months!

What a huge relief it was for me to see Apollo actually wandering around in the yard without any help, having the most normal movement I had seen since before he broke his leg. It was more than I could have possibly asked for, it was a miracle.

I sent Doc a fax to let him know how well Apollo was doing. Apollo was home within hours and Apollo woke up the next day as if nothing had happened. I was one very appreciative and grateful owner, so many of my prayers had been answered, a much greater spirit was looking after Apollo. I was not questioning at that point. I was only very thankful.

I felt from that point as if I would only observe Apollo getting better and better. I wondered why I had not removed his leg sooner? I felt like I had not betrayed my friend after all by amputating his leg.

The next few days Apollo did terrific, he was up and about on and off the deck and seemed like he felt great!

I decided our new "opportunity" (as I began to call our challenges) was to figure out how to modify Apollo's walkabout so that he could go for walks without tiring himself out. The walk about was made for dogs with four legs, it just did not work for a three-legged dog. That Sunday I went to the home improvement store in search of something to help modify the walk about. I was very determined to come up with something to "modify the walk-about harness" so that Apollo could go for at least a couple of short walks a day. I did finally adapt the walk about and Apollo soon was able to go for a couple of little walks each day. It was actually less work for Apollo than it was for Joe or me; he used his front legs and we supported his back legs. Although, he didn't have any idea that was the case, we had the real "workouts" for each walk.

Apollo didn't know he had cancer. He didn't know he had his leg removed. He did not know he a bald hip, shaved for his surgery. What Apollo did know was that he was surrounded by unconditional love and he had a love of life, he wanted to continue - and his enthusiasm, his spirit showed it.

Chapter 14

The Big Blizzard!

Apollo was doing very well and then we experienced another "opportunity." It was only the end of October and we were lucky enough to be hit with an early blizzard. It was truly a big blizzard and the first to hit Denver in several years. I was actually okay with early snow, it meant Joe couldn't make it in to work the next day and neither could anyone else in Denver, a real snow day!

The snow kept falling and falling. Our greatest challenge was to keep up with shoveling the snow off our back yard deck just to make it easy for Apollo to get out the door and outside when he needed to.

After about twenty-five inches of snow had fallen, it finally stopped snowing and the scene was beautiful. I remember thinking about how amazing it was for Apollo to enjoy this-another season of snow, after all, he was not even supposed to live more than three or four months after he was diagnosed with osteosarcoma. Yet Apollo was alive 11 months later, without any chemotherapy. *He had defied the odds.* Apollo seemed even more amazing and I continued to treasure our time together.

The next day it was then time for us to tackle the driveway and front sidewalk and do more shoveling. Joe and I both went out early the next morning to shovel the front driveway and sidewalk. Apollo sat in the living room, looked out the front window watching us. He began barking at us, that was unusual for Apollo. He really wanted to come outside and be with us. After some hesitation and shoveling almost an entire path we let Apollo outside with us. He actually pulled us in the snow. Apollo wanted to go visit every neighbor and dog.

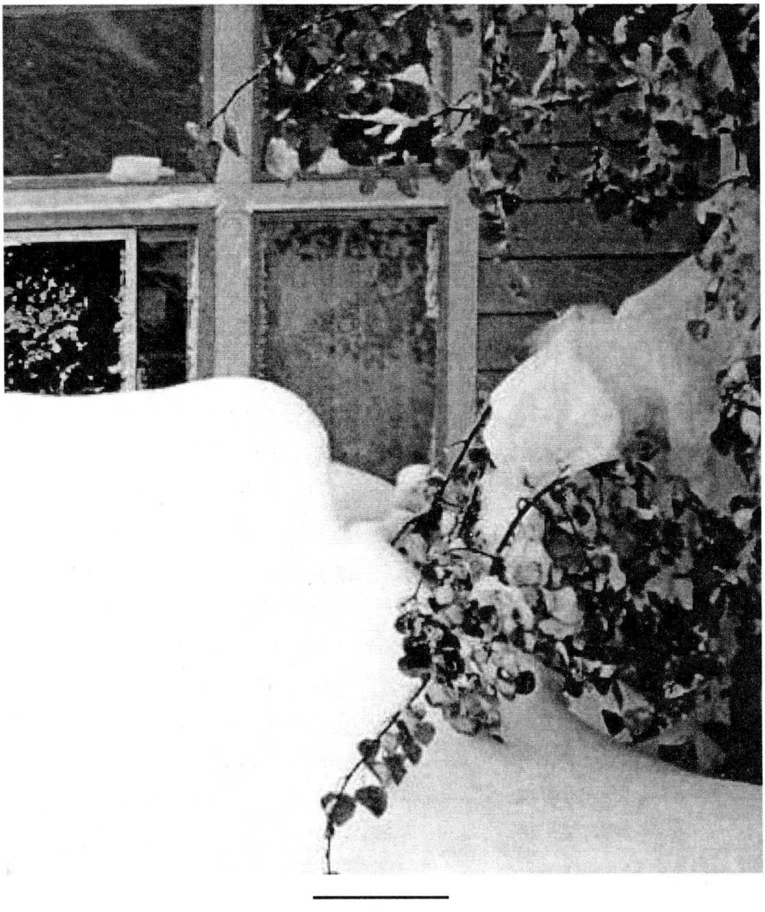

Apollo loved being out in the snow and he lay down and rolled his face in the snow just as he always had. It was wonderful to see. After Apollo had had his romp in the snow, we took him inside and did our warm-up routine - hot soup, moist heating pad and a thick, comfy big, warm blanket. My puppy dog was happy and enjoyed being a snow dog once again. Watching Apollo's reaction to the snow and him really wanting to go play in the white sutff was huge encouragement to me. I felt that he had so much spirit and determination to keep on living even with only three legs he had adapted. He was once again living up to be the fighter he was named after - Apollo Creed.

Chapter 15

Apollo & Me
Our Last Few Weeks Together

On Sunday, November 2nd, I told Joe I thought Apollo was hurting. Apollo didn't really want to move around too much, he was lying around and every once in a while, he would let out kind of a whining sound. I tried the things I thought had worked before...the moist heating pad, and the warm soup. The only thing that really seemed to help was snuggling up to him and giving him a nice massage.

It reminded me of his first nights with me as a puppy. I think Apollo had me very well trained. As long as he was getting his massage he was fine. If I stopped, however, he began to whine again. Apollo and I made a trip that Sunday afternoon to Aspen Park, I just couldn't let him whine...something was hurting him and I had to find out what.

When we arrived Apollo was examined; we checked his temperature, which was normal, we could not see anything wrong with him. The physical examination didn't look like he had any broken bones. We scheduled an appointment to go back again the next day and my pup came home with an aspirin/muscle relaxant combination and temaril.

It was terribly cold outside and I thought maybe Apollo's spinal spondolosis was causing him the discomfort. He had that condition since he was about two and a half years old. I hoped that was what was causing him to whine.

The combination of medications had relieved Apollo's pain a little, but he was still hurting, so on November 13, we returned again to Aspen Park and had x-rays taken. Apollo's lungs, liver, pancreas and spleen all looked clear! His left back leg also looked

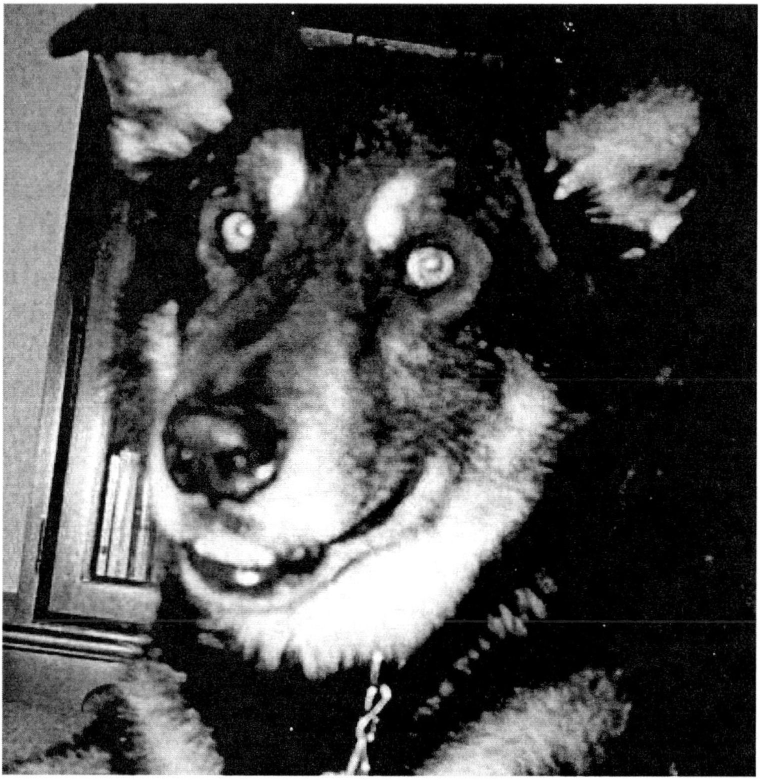

fine, no broken bones. The only thing apparent on the x-rays was the spinal spondolosis. This was really a GREAT day, from what we could see Apollo's cancer had not metastasized! It was 11 months to the day that Apollo had broken his leg; I couldn't have asked for more. I had the gift of more time than I had imagined with my little puppy dog. This was another day for celebration!

Now, if only we could relieve the discomfort the spondolosis was causing. I recalled thinking to myself; "This was just another bump in the road," and I left Doc's office that day, scheduling appointments for November 18 and 25. I distinctly remember telling Apollo as we drove home ,"Apollo you will be with me for the holidays ...and we will make them the best ever for you!" This was just another little challenge and I knew we could "fix it," somehow we could make Apollo feel really good again.

Since the cancer had not spread to any other organs I considered this situation to be a "big old dog" syndrome and what a relief. After all we had been through, I felt Apollo and I could easily handle this new situation. I promised Apollo we would stop whatever was hurting. Apollo had his acupuncture and he felt better by the time we arrived back at home, in fact he wanted to stay out in the front yard and observe everything that was going on in the neighborhood.

Chapter 16

Our Final Farewell... But I am Not Ready to Say Goodbye Yet

About one week before Apollo left forever; I was concerned that he was having difficultly being able getting up and around. He was doing somewhat better, but still seemed to be in some pain. I snuggled up next to him often, scratching his chest. I told him over and over "Apollo... tell me what is wrong, your bum leg is gone, you don't have cancer in your lungs and I want to fix what is making you hurt, but I don't know what is hurting you now." I was searching for answers... the feeling of helplessness once again returned.

I had planned to be working out of town all day on November 19, and also until very late afternoon on the November 20. Joe had planned on taking off about noon that day since I was going to be home late, and we did not want Apollo to be alone for more than three to four hours until we knew he was able to move around the house without difficulty. I called Doc's office to see if perhaps I could bring Apollo up early on the 19th for "Doggie Day Care" and observation. I thought it would be great for Apollo to be at his second home and also this would give Doc the opportunity to observe Apollo for a longer period of time to determine how we could maybe get over this recent "bump in the road. "

I also made contingency plans in case we had a terrible snow and I couldn't get Apollo to Aspen Park because of bad weather. Apollo and I checked on B&B for DOGS, as an alternative if we needed one. There, Apollo would have remained in the company of the other geriatric dogs. Just knowing that Apollo wouldn't be left alone at home, no matter what, gave me great comfort.

On the evening of the 18th as I prepared Apollo's treats and ice cubes for his bedtime snack, I debated leaving him down stairs, because I knew we would be up very early in order to be in Aspen Park by 7:30 the next morning.

Apollo sat at the bottom of the stairs looked at me tilting his head from side to side as if to say, "I want to go upstairs and be with you." Of course, if Apollo wanted to be with me, I couldn't resist, so with some help from me, Apollo went upstairs to sleep at the foot of the bed. I ran downstairs and fixed another bowl of ice cubes, dog treats and took those up to him, thinking he deserved a few extras for his effort in getting upstairs. As usual before turning the lights out, I gave Apollo a huge hug and kiss; I told him he was the best dog in the world. I had no idea at that time that would be our last night together...forever. I am so grateful that I paid attention to what Apollo wanted rather than what I thought would be most convenient for me.

The following morning, November 19, I awoke at 5:00 a.m. so that I could get ready for work, before waking Apollo up and helping him downstairs. When it was time to leave, I gave Apollo a little extra time to stretch before I helped him walk downstairs. He got up feeling better than I had seen him feel in the last week and I remember thinking, "I sure am glad that you wanted to go upstairs to be with me last night Apollo."

We walked around the front yard for a while and I was so relieved that he seemed much more comfortable than he had in a long time.

During our drive to Aspen Park, Apollo seemed alert and happy to be going for a ride. He had his head out the window and also looked for the horses as we neared Doc's office. I even told him, "Apollo, you are a spoiled dog! I am probably being foolish to not leave you alone at home today, you would probably be just fine."

When we arrived at Aspen Park, Apollo got out of the car. He wanted to keep walking around outside, I was thrilled to see him feeling good. I thought to myself, "We have just been through another little rough spot."

Doc told me he was planning on closely observing Apollo throughout the day. I left knowing that Apollo was in the finest hands and he would have a lot of attention and love while I worked that day. I told everyone that I would be back to pick Apollo up between 5:30 and 6:00 p.m. that evening and Apollo was very happy and comfortable in Doc's office.

I remember leaving Apollo with one of Doc's technician's, hugged Apollo and her giving him lots of attention. I told Apollo that I would be "right back." For the first time in so many numerous trips to Aspen Park, I NEVER considered that Apollo would not come home with me that evening. Maybe that was another gift… for both Apollo and me. Apollo and I could have never told one another goodbye, he stayed for me and I was there forever for him- my best friend. I left knowing that no matter how inconvenient, no matter how foolish, I had done what I thought was best for Apollo. I called Joe as I was driving back to Denver and told him I was planning on both of us being home by 7:00 p.m. that evening.

As I waited for my manager to arrive at Denver International Airport around 9:15 a.m., I ran into my neighbor and friend who was also in the medical field and knew of Apollo's battle for life. He asked me about Apollo. I proceeded to tell him about this amazing miracle, acupuncture, massage, vitamins, shark cartlidge, colloidial minerals and even reiki treatments and that I had just left Apollo for a stay at Aspen Park for "doggie day care."

I talked about the health care options we had available. These were choices not based on what insurance would cover…I did not have pet health care insurance for Apollo. These were not choices based on what "managed care" insurance allowed me to do. All of the treatments were based on what I thought was the very latest and best in medical care available to Apollo. All of what I had chosen to do was based on what would provide Apollo the best quality of life, regardless of how long that timeframe was. I remember telling my friend, "If nothing else, I know Apollo has had the very best. You and I could have had no better medical care than Apollo has had."

I finished my day at about 5:15 p.m. and I called Aspen Park to let them know it would be closer to 6:00 p.m. before I would be there. I didn't want to keep anyone too late. For a second, I thought about leaving Apollo overnight but I really wanted to have him home with us and I was anxious to hear what Doc's observation had concluded.

When I arrived in Aspen Park, I was relieved to see that Doc was still seeing patients and I started walking to the back office to find Apollo. The front office told me to go back to surgery, where Apollo was often treated. When Apollo wasn't in surgery I looked in Doc's office...no Apollo, so I looked in the lab-another one of Apollo's regular hangout spots at the clinic.

I called for Apollo and I heard him whine and saw him on a bed of soft, fluffy pillows and blankets in the laboratory. My first thought was that he must have had a day of too much play, after all that morning he seemed very frisky. As Apollo tried to get up he cried, so I sat on the floor with him scratching his chest and telling him we would once again fix "it " whatever "it" was.

Doc then came into the lab and told me he had something to show me. We walked back into an exam room to view an x-ray and I saw it...Apollo had broken his front left leg.

Doc said Apollo had gone for a walk in the early afternoon, everything seemed to be fine, and then about 4:00 he was lying down and tried to get up... he was interested in what another dog was up to... the bone just snapped. It was a spiral fracture.

My tears began to flow uncontrollably... for almost the past year, my biggest fear was that Apollo would break another bone. I promised Apollo that if he ever did, I would not make him suffer through another broken bone. Yet I had to ask... I had to try and see if there was anything else we could do. Doc told me we could do surgery... plates and screws, but from the x-rays Apollo's other front leg appeared to be very thin and brittle, it might break too. The x-rays showed the very brittle bones.

Apollo was an old dog for as big as he was. He was still my puppy dog... the cute shy little puppy who had stolen my heart. This was too soon; I was just not ready to say goodbye. We still had walks to take; we still had another trip to The Little Nell... Apollo still had treats at home, he had not even finished eating. I was not ready to say goodbye, but then I had always said I never would be. This was not about me, this was about Apollo and I had to keep my promise to Apollo, I knew there really wasn't any choice...it was time to say goodbye.

But how do you tell your best friend goodbye?

Even though Apollo had lived eight to nine months longer than anyone expected, I still felt this was not enough time together. But, I always knew that no matter how much time I had with Apollo, I would *never* be ready to say goodbye. I think that I was very lucky to have had such a good friend, he was always there for me and now it was time for me to be strong and be there for him.

I looked at the clock... it was 6:20 p.m. November 19 and Joe was somewhere in rush hour traffic and probably wouldn't be home for another half-hour. If

I waited for Joe it would have been at least 8:00 p.m. before he could be in Aspen Park with us.

Apollo was in pain and I also didn't want to keep Doc and his staff that late even though they were very supportive and told me over and over to take my time. This time I knew…there was no point in praying for some more time…I had prayed and begged for more time and our time was up. I knew in my heart there were to be no more miracles, we had already been given the gift of many miracles… our life together as we knew it was about to be change forever.

I finally had to concede that I had done absolutely everything I could possibly do for Apollo. Apollo had fought his battle against cancer as hard and for as long as he could and that battle was finally almost over. I had to believe that as hard as it was for me, it was Apollo's time to leave for good. It was time for him to move on and I needed to let him go. I needed to be very strong for Apollo at that moment.

I sat on the floor with Apollo and I felt so helpless, even though he had some painkillers, he cried when he tried to move. I couldn't even lie down and snuggle up with him to scratch his favorite spot on his chest because I was afraid I would hurt him, so I sat in front of him scratching his chest. I asked Apollo to give me a kiss and he licked and licked my face. I knew I just couldn't make him wait for Joe. I rubbed between Apollo's toes; Joe would have done the same for Apollo. I had always wanted to have Apollo put to sleep at home, but we could not have moved him without making him hurt even more, and Doc's office and everyone there had become Apollo's second home and family. I knew that we had only a few moments left at best and even those were stolen moments. Apollo had been here and beaten the odds but it was so obvious he could no longer fight.

My main objective in saying goodbye to Apollo had always been to make his final journey as peaceful and loving as possible. I knew that I didn't want Apollo hearing me wail and sob. I knew that the only things I wanted Apollo to feel was that I was there with him, to love and take care of him. I also knew that I didn't want him to be in pain much longer and he had broken his leg about two hours earlier.

While I was so grateful that Doc and his staff had waited for me to get there, I didn't want Apollo hurting any longer because of my selfishness. I spent about 15 minutes longer scratching Apollo's chest, petting his head, kissing him softly and telling him over and over in a calm, soothing voice, "I am right here with you Apollo, just relax, relax we are going to fix this now, no more hurting…you are the best dog Apollo, so you just rest now and I will take care of you. I love you and I am right here with you big dog." I told Doc that we were ready…ready as we could ever be, it was time…

Doc gave Apollo a sedative. He said that would take about 10 minutes or so to take effect. Then when that had taken effect he would administer another injection interveinously and that would cause everything to stop. Apollo became very sleepy and Doc's staff carried him into another exam room and gently put him on the exam table. He was then given an injection which would result in Apollo's his peaceful transistion. His "opportunities" would be over. In a blur of tears, while remaining with him, I had to make the decision to let him go. I knew there was not any other choice for Apollo. I signed all of the paperwork...I never read anything. I knew I trusted the hands we were in. One of Doc's technicians asked me if I wanted Apollo cremated, which I knew I did. I still kept speaking softly to him...I wanted him to hear my voice, feel my touch and know that I was still there with him. There was never any question in my mind that I would remain with my best friend until the very last moment he left forever.

Doc checked Apollo's heart and said Apollo had taken his final journey home. While still telling Apollo I loved him and he was the best dog, I held his paw in my hand and kissed him goodbye. As gut-wrenching as it was, it was the last act of love and kindness I could do for my beloved dog. Any other decision would have been cruel.

I stayed with Apollo for a while. The technicians sheared some fur from Apollo's chest and gave me Apollo's bright red collar. I then had a few minutes alone to hug Apollo for the last time. I couldn't tell Apollo goodbye. Goodbye to me seemed so definite, it seemed like there wouldn't be anything left. Apollo had given me so much, he taught me more about life and love than anyone else could ever have. He was always the teacher, the master and the gifts I received, and the lessons I have learned will always be with me. In many ways, Apollo will always be with me.

One of the things I remember Doc telling me was that the hardest part of this would be the emptiness...

the big hole. That emptiness felt more like the Grand Canyon than a big hole. However as hard as it was to say goodbye forever to my best friend. I also felt so very lucky. I was able to be with Apollo as he journeyed from this life, as he knew it. I felt as if I were able to accompany him from one journey to the next with only love and peacefulness leading the way.

He was never alone as I had never been alone since he had come into my life. As so terribly hard it was I would be eternally grateful I was fortunate enough to be with Apollo for 10 years and also during the last moments of his life. I feel that he left this earth with no fear, no panic, no bitterness and no anger, after all he had been through. I truly believe he only felt love. He exited this world in the same way he entered it with innocence and unconditional love.

I believe that my Grand Canyon was not meant to be filled, but rather treasured forever.

Apollo, every moment truly was a gift and I thank you my puppy dog for all of your unconditional love, companionship and guidance in the true meaning of life. You were absolutely my very best friend and no matter what else there is, I will always have the most special place in my heart for you and I will always miss you. Thank you and farewell my Apollo, until we meet again.

Chapter 17

My Doggie is Gone… Dealing With the Emptiness

When I left Doc and Aspen Park I did not know how I would drive home. Joe had told one of Doc's technician's that he would come and get me, however I thought it wouldn't be practical to have two vehicles 37 miles away from home. I knew could make it home. I had Apollo as an angel on my shoulder. He still be guided me. However still with unstoppable tears, I did not know how I could ever be without Apollo again.

The night Apollo left my life forever, I went home in tears to Joe and all I could say was "my puppy dog is gone." Our tears flowed as we held each other, even though we had had known Apollo probably would not be here for several more years, even though I had had time to prepare I just was not ready to say goodbye to Apollo. We had had several "close calls" over the year I was just not ready to give up on Apollo as long as he was happy and had a good quality of life. I believe there was definitely a greater ***spirit*** looking out for us. The situation with Apollo's newly broken leg left Apollo and I no other choice.

One of the things, which was the hardest, was never being sure when and how I would say my final goodbye. I really wanted Apollo to be put to sleep at our home, but I also knew that would be very hard, knowing that I would choose the day he would leave forever. So, in retrospect I believe as difficult as it was to make the decision to finally let go we were given a gift, after all we had been through it was out of our hands.

That night, I hardly slept and could hardly breathe through all of the tears, we cried not for Apollo, but for our loss. We talked about some of our trips with Apollo, our nightly walks with Apollo, our just being with Apollo. All we really ever gave was our care and love and in return Apollo loved us and taught us that one of the most important things in life *is* caring and giving love.

We talked about the hardest part of Apollo's death was that he just wouldn't be with us and this feeling came up over and over again.

Joe was used to coming home each night and finding Apollo waiting for him at the door, Apollo would nuzzle right up to Joe for some immediate attention. The thing I missed most was hugging Apollo; he was so huggable and I almost never walked by him without just giving him a big hug.

That Christmas was extremely difficult. For nine years, I never went to get a Christmas tree without Apollo. He always seemed to like walking around the tree lot with me maybe he just liked all the attention he got, anyway getting a tree without him was very hard. He used to also sit in the front yard with me when I put the lights up, I considered not doing lights that year, but Apollo showed so much strength even when I thought he would have not wanted to be bothered. He was my inspiration to continue with the tradition of putting the lights up again that year. I also hung Apollo's Christmas stocking and put one of his partially eaten rawhide bones in it. On Christmas day, Joe and I toasted to Apollo, for he is still with us in our thoughts and in our hearts and he always will be.

A few weeks later I received the call I wanted; yet I dreaded…Apollo's ashes were back. It was late afternoon when I received the message, so I knew where I would be the next morning. It seems the longest drive ever was the drive to Aspen Park to pick up Apollo's remains. I didn't notice the sunrise on that morning trip. Somehow picking up Apollo's ashes made everything seem so much more final. I thought at first the days right after Apollo died would be the worst, but I now realized that as time has passed, Apollo and I were never separated for more than 10 days and only a few times in our 10 years. That is why on some days it just seemed so empty without him.

On my drive home, I felt some comfort knowing that Apollo's remains would always be with me and I decided to stop and get some flowers to put with his urn of ashes. I purchased three long-stemmed yellow roses, baby's breath and a red bow. Yellow roses are for friendship and that seemed very fitting for my best friend. I believe that it helped to do whatever I could to find comfort in. Joe placed Apollo's red collar in our curio cabinet among toasting goblets and each time I pass by I am able to smile. I think Apollo always knew he was a treasure in my life.

I also believe that it is *okay to grieve*. I think it would be unhealthy to not allow myself to do that. Some days are BIG missing Apollo days and some days I was able to just remember the great times we had, and know that Apollo's challenges are over. I think of his amazing strength and gentleness. Throughout his entire last year of life, with all of the injections, bandages, poking and prodding he never once growled or showed his teeth. He trusted and knew I was just doing whatever I needed to do to take care of him.

It is because I did do everything I could to make Apollo feel well and I did what I thought was in his best interest without giving up on him. I can truly say I don't have any regrets...he always had the best. I could have done no less for my very best friend.

My Letter to Apollo

Dear Apollo,

So how do I tell my best friend goodbye? I have sat holding your collar and leash and I cried and cried. I cried for more time with you because we did not have enough time together, and even though we had more time than anyone expected us to have, it was still not enough. You have been my constant companion, my inspiration and my best friend and I don't know what I will do without you. Maybe I shouldn't be so sad; maybe you have left to move on and share your gifts in some other ways. You brought much love and happiness to my life, I was very fortunate. It is true that dog is God spelled backwards, I just wished that God had made dogs live forever.

I am always going to miss you my big dog, I promised you I would not keep you here and make you suffer, so I had to let you go. I did everything I could. I know you did everything you could and we had no choice; our time together was over. Joe said that you stayed for an encore, but all encore's still have to come to an end, I never wanted yours to end. In spite of the rocky road we have traveled together over the last year, I would not change a thing. Wherever you are now, Apollo, I am blowing you a kiss and throwing you a big hug and I hope that you are enjoying a big bowl of ice cubes and treats. I will always miss you my big dog, every moment with you was truly a gift.

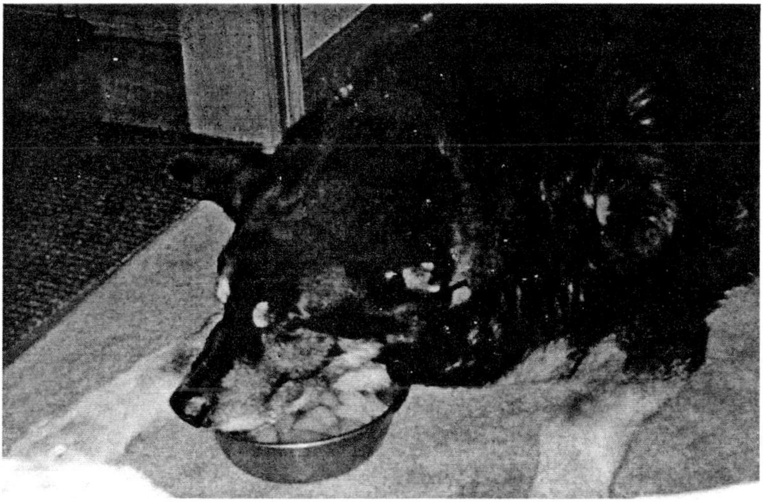

Why I Wrote Apollo's Creed

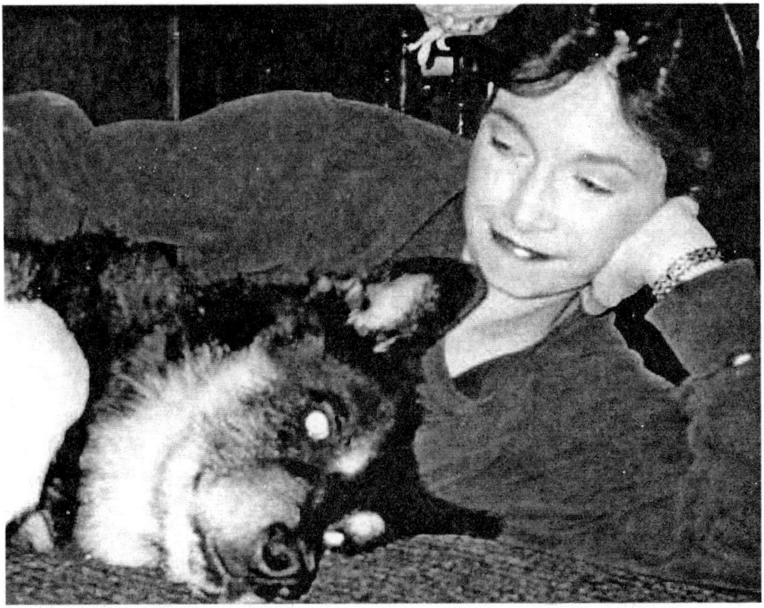

When Apollo and I were going through this ordeal, I couldn't find any resource - book or otherwise - to help me make these hard decisions. So, I created the book that I wished I could have found then. As Apollo and I took this journey together, I searched for answers and the only place I could find them was in my heart. This book is for you - first, to know you're not alone facing this - and second to be a source of pertinent information and true comfort during this difficult time.

Apollo lasted eleven months longer than anyone expected, so each and every day, I questioned my intentions. "Was I honoring him as a living being by trying to extend his life (and quality of life) by trying all of these traditional, alternative and cutting edge options? Did he really want this? Would I have wanted someone to do this for me?"

Some people say I pushed the envelope too far, but I knew my dog, so I was at peace.

This book is intended to give you permission to listen - not only to your vet - but to your heart and to your dog, when you have to make these difficult decisions.

I used my medical background as a bridge and I took good notes throughout the ordeal, so that I could tell the story that would not only honor Apollo, but your pet as well.

I hope this book serves as a resource to assist you on your path. I wish you peace and above all - no regrets!

~ Deb Estes

So many days have passed and yet
The memory remains.
And still of soft and silent nights
You come to us again

We see you as we knew you once:
You seem to smile, and then,
We see ourselves there at your side
As often it had been.

And we return the smile you give
And cherish in our hearts
The thought that we had days to share
Before we had to part.

And we find that time has not erased,
Nor has its passages paled,
That warmth we held for you in life;
That love has not failed.

And so dear friend, we keep you close,
Although we are apart,
And with you daily in
The visions of our hearts.

~Author Unkown

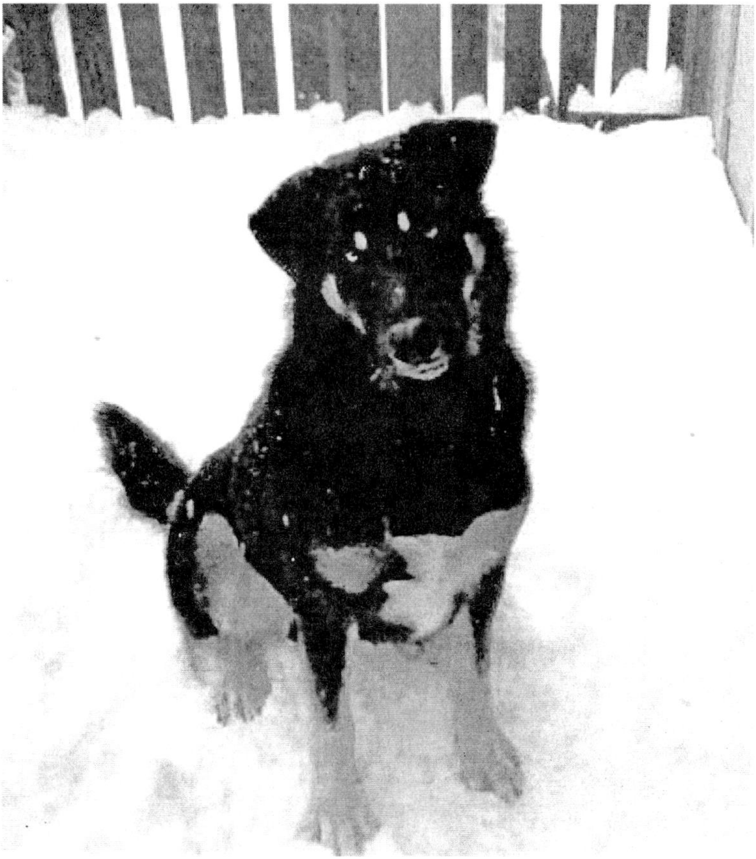

To order copies of the book

APOLLO'S CREED

$19.97 + 2.50(S&H)

online at:
www.BooksToBelieveIn.com/ApollosCreed.php

by phone:
(call for volume discounts)
(303) 794-8888

by fax:
(720) 863-2013

by mail: send check payable to:
Thornton Publishing, Inc.
17011 Lincoln Ave. #408
Parker, Colorado 80134

If it is temporarily sold out at your favorite bookstore, have them order more of **ISBN: 0-9779960-8-5**

Name: ______________________________
Address: ______________________________
____

Phone: ______________________________
E-mail: ______________________________

Credit Card #: ______________________________
Card Type: ______________ Expiration Date: ___/___
Security Code: ________